Dr Eva Orsmond's 10lb Diet

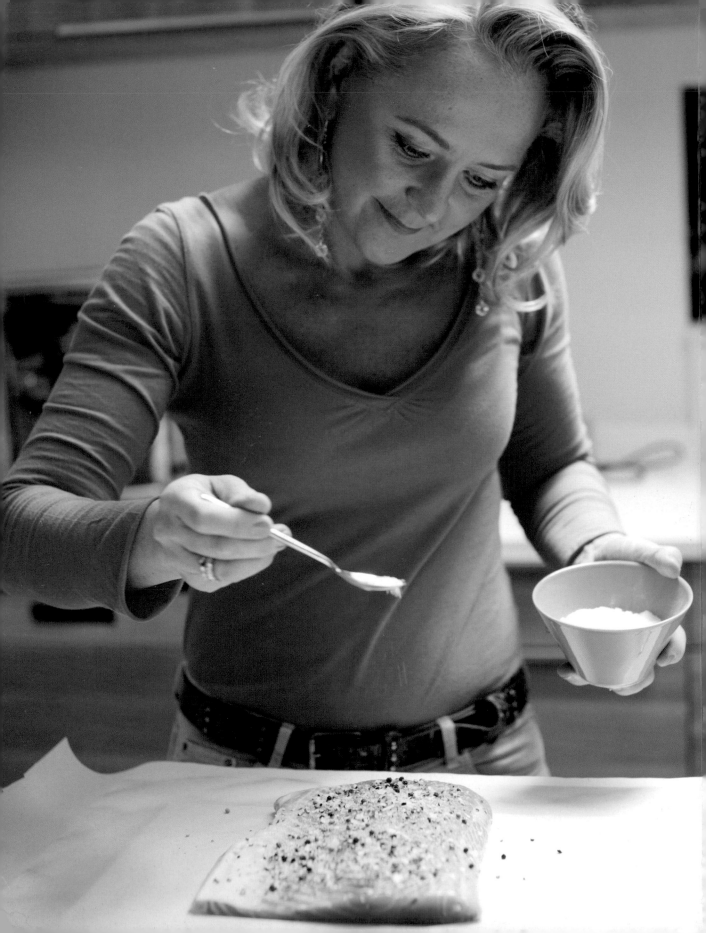

Dr Eva Orsmond's

10LB
DIET

A Fast Plan
A Slow Plan
A New You

GILL & MACMILLAN

Gill & Macmillan
Hume Avenue
Park West
Dublin 12

with associated companies throughout the world
www.gillmacmillanbooks.ie

ISBN: 978 07171 60099

Designed by www.grahamthew.com
Edited by Dog's-ear
Photography by Hugh McElveen
Food styling by Gwynne Searle
Props supplied by Brown Thomas, House of Fraser and Meadows & Byrne
Hair styling by Annie at Profile Hair Design
Indexed by Jane Rogers
Printed by Printer Trento Srl, Italy

This book is typeset in Dederon Derif 9pt on 11 pt.
The paper used in this book comes from the wood pulp of managed forests.
For every tree felled, at least one is planted, thereby renewing natural resources.

A catalogue record for this book is available from the British Library.
5432

Contents

Acknowledgements viii

INTRODUCTION
What 10lb will do for you 4
Analyse your lifestyle 6
Motivate yourself 8

THE PLANS
How to use the plans 10
The Fast Plan: 10lb in 3 weeks 12
The Slow Plan: 10lb in 12 weeks 14
Exercise plan 16
Diet diaries 22

THE RECIPES
BREAKFAST
Dr Eva's Eggs Benedict 34
Barley Porridge (Ohraryynipuuro) 37
Skagen 38
Banana Pancake 40
Courgette and Bacon Pancake 41
Cauliflower Scrambled Eggs 44
Buckwheat Flatbreads 45
Raspberry Smoothie 46
Scrambled Eggs with Caviar 48
Finnish Whipped Porridge (Vispipuuro) 51
Purple 'Pick Me Up' Juice 52

LUNCH
Dill-Cured Salmon Tartare 58
Seafood Rice Paper Rolls 60
Spinach and Feta Quesadilla 63

FILLER SOUPS
Summer Soup 64
Mima's Cabbage Soup 66
Tom Yum Soup 67
Celeriac Mushroom Soup 71
Tomato Soup 72
Pea and Mint Soup 75
Celery Roquefort Soup 76
Thai Mushroom Soup 78
Tricolour Soup 79

SOUPS AS A MEAL

Borscht **81**
Creamy Chorizo Soup **83**
Russian Soup (Solyanka) **84**
Pork Sausage Soup (Siskonmakkarakeitto) **87**
Fish Soup **88**
Chinese Chicken Soup **90**
Leek and Potato Soup **91**

Waldorf Salad **95**
Warm Halloumi Salad **96**
Tex-Mex Salad **98**
Sushi Salad **100**
Seafood Salad **103**

DINNER

Cowboy Stew **106**
Pomegranate and Beef Casserole **108**
Lamb Rogan Josh **111**
Stuffed Onions **112**
Turkish Pizza **114**
Farmer's Pie **116**
Bacon and Halloumi Stew **117**

Fish Rolls **121**
Portuguese Squid **123**
Easy Fish Pie **124**
Creamy Prawn Risotto **125**
Prawn Stir-Fry **126**
Fish with Mushroom Sauce **128**
Baked Trout **129**

Turkey Burgers with Celeriac Chips **130**
Spicy Chicken Tacos **133**
Chicken Fried Rice **134**
Turkey Meatballs in Tomato Sauce **135**
Chicken Kebabs with Pomegranate Molasses **139**
Chicken Tikka Masala **140**
Chicken Butternut Bake **142**

Fried Halloumi and Cumin-Spiced Leeks 145
Vegetarian Sausage Stew 146
Sweet and Sour Stir-Fry 147
Yellow Dal 149
Vegetable Fajitas 150
Vegetable Green Curry 152
Courgette Bake 154
Turnip and Celeriac Bake 155

'Now to Wow' Lasagne 157
Chilli Pasta Bolognese 158
Easy Cauliflower Carbonara 161
Creamy Ham and Garlic Pasta 162

SNACKS, SIDES AND DRINKS

Great Grandma's Berry Soup (Kiisseli) 166
Coconut Biscuits 169
Carrot and Beetroot Muffins 170
Granola Protein Bars 173
Ultimate Health Loaf 174
Crudités with Dips 176
Finnish Pâté (Maksapasteija) 179
Smoked Mackerel Pâté 180
Creamy Salmon Pâté 180
Baba Ganoush 181
Cauliflower Mash 184
Pak Choi Stir-Fry 187
Courgette Hummus 188
High Fibre Salad 189
Mustard and Anchovy Dressing 192
Ginger Garlic Paste 195
Mustard 196
Mayonnaise 196

Earl Grey Iced Tea with Mint 199
Rooibos and Apple Iced Tea 200
White Wine Sangria 203
Hot Chocolate 204
Italian-Style Coffee 207

Unusual ingredients 208
Index 210

Acknowledgements

You are holding my second book in your hand. It was a challenge to choose and tweak my favourite recipes gathered from my childhood in Finland and university time in Italy. This book is a combination of efforts: it would never have seen the daylight without the support, hard work and patience of many people.

I want to thank Fergal and Nicki at Gill & Macmillan who believed in me and pushed me so that I could respect the tight deadlines to get this book done.

My amazing staff, especially Katri and Marie, have been with me through the 'thick and thin' to get all the final details sorted.

For Emma and Ronan, I have a special word: you two are responsible for the readable version of this book. You don't have any limits to your patience and hard work. It must be because you are living in sunny France. You must be drinking wine every hour of the day to keep you so cool and relaxed!!

Last but not least, my dear family. Thanks to my mother, Kirsti-Mima, who collected and organised props from Finnish designers to keep the Finnish design style in the pictures – and of course for her amazing ideas for recipes. To my son Evan, who had to listen to my panicked outbursts before the tight deadlines and who gave me love when I needed it. To my son Chris – thank you for eating all this low calorie food when in reality you needed more substantial food to keep your rugby body moving. To my dear husband, Wyatt: thank you for your long emails while sailing the world seas and thank you for loving me. But this time you do not get credit for the book! To dear Gabi, thank you for always being there! And dear Hugh and my sister-in-law Gwynne – you did a fantastic job. THANK YOU.

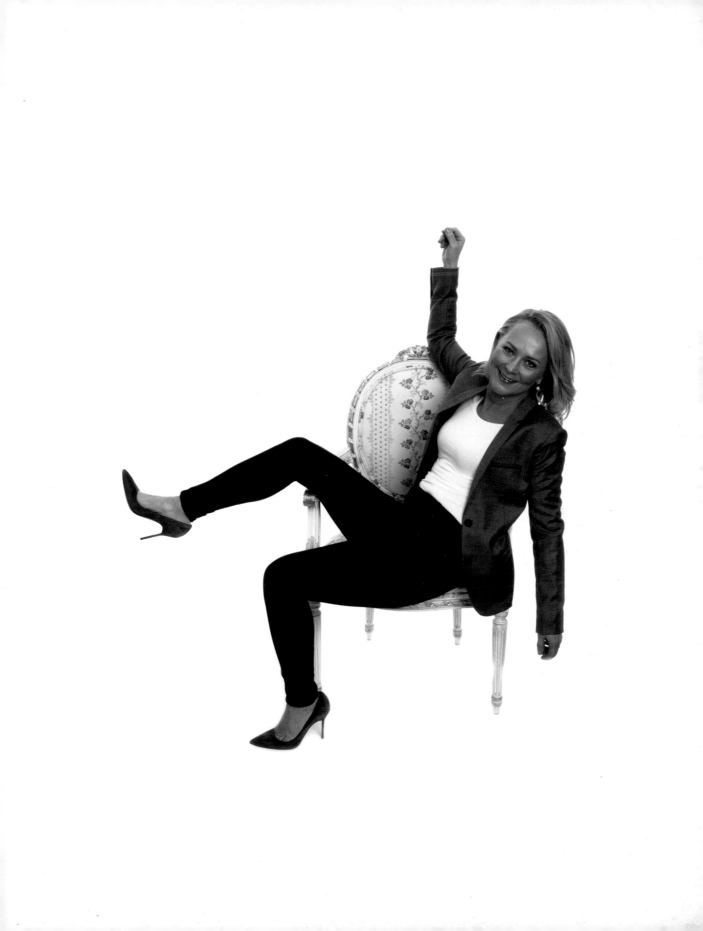

Diet is the foundation of good health. If you ask your doctor or dietician what you should eat, they usually recommend a 'balanced diet'. But what is the right balanced diet for you?

People hear so much conflicting information that they are more uncertain than ever before. They are so keen to feel better and they want to find the right diet that will solve their problems – everything from intermittent fasting, alkaline diet, caveman diet, organic diet, dairy-free diet or low-carb diet. They try all the trends but they become confused.

We want to talk about food all of the time, we want to eat all of the time – and yet we do not want to *think* about food! In our society, we do not think clearly about what we are eating or how much we are eating!

The reality is this: many people have major problems in their diets. Every day, I meet people who are suffering from irritable bowel, bloating, heartburn, thinning hair, cracked nails, itchy skin, stiff joints, headaches, infertility, excess hair, insomnia, mood swings, low energy – the list is endless!

Over the last 12 years, I have helped many people to overcome these problems: to feel better and to look better. All of this has been done by concentrating on people's diets. I believe that many health problems are preventable. I do not recommend magic pills or quick fixes: I believe in better lifestyle choices.

But before you get to the better lifestyle, you must look at your lifestyle today. You must stop and think about things. Stop here and now. Stop being in denial! Ask yourself the important questions. Do you have health problems? Could you improve your diet? Would you feel better if you lost some weight?

As I know what a difference 4.5kg (10lb) does for me and my patients, I am sharing with you my 10lb Diet. I hope it will give you the 'wow factor' to get you to your best place and to motivate you to challenge yourself more. By the time you have read this book, you will know me better and you will know what I think is the secret to a healthier, younger you! I hope from the bottom of my heart that you enjoy what I have planned for you.

With love
Con amore
Rakkaudella

Dr Eva

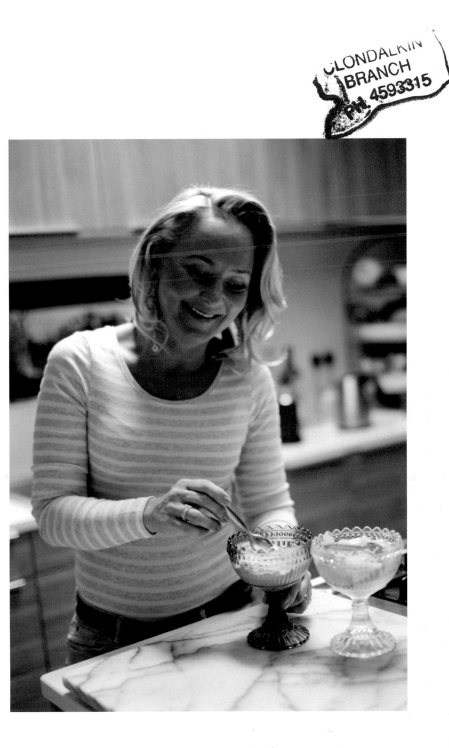

The 10lb Diet is about making a simple commitment that will create huge gains for your health, looks and wellbeing. Of course, 10lb means different things to different people.

Maybe if you are very overweight, you think that 10lb won't make a difference. But I always say: 'Any weightloss is better than no weightloss!' If you have a lot of weight to lose, then losing the first 10lb will teach you how to have a healthier lifestyle. What is more, losing 10lb now will give you all the motivation you need to lose even more weight in the future.

Maybe you are not very overweight – but this can be very hard to judge nowadays. Unfortunately, many people underestimate the amount of weight they are actually carrying. Overweight is the new normal! But even if you do not have much weight to lose, the 10lb Diet will help you to 'clean up your act'. My patients say to me all the time that losing 10lb really does make a difference. If you lose 10lb, there are many things you can look forward to. You can:

- Lower your risk of high blood pressure and cholesterol, diabetes and prediabetes, stroke and cancer

- Improve your digestion: reduce IBS, bloating, cramps and heartburn

- Boost your brain power and concentration

- Stabilise your hormones and boost your libido

- Help your immune system

- Regulate your appetite: keep the hunger pangs at bay

- Reduce stress

- Improve your mood

- Enjoy restful sleep

- Age more gracefully

- Feel slim and comfortable in your clothes

- Enjoy glowing skin, shiny hair and strong nails

- Feel more energetic!

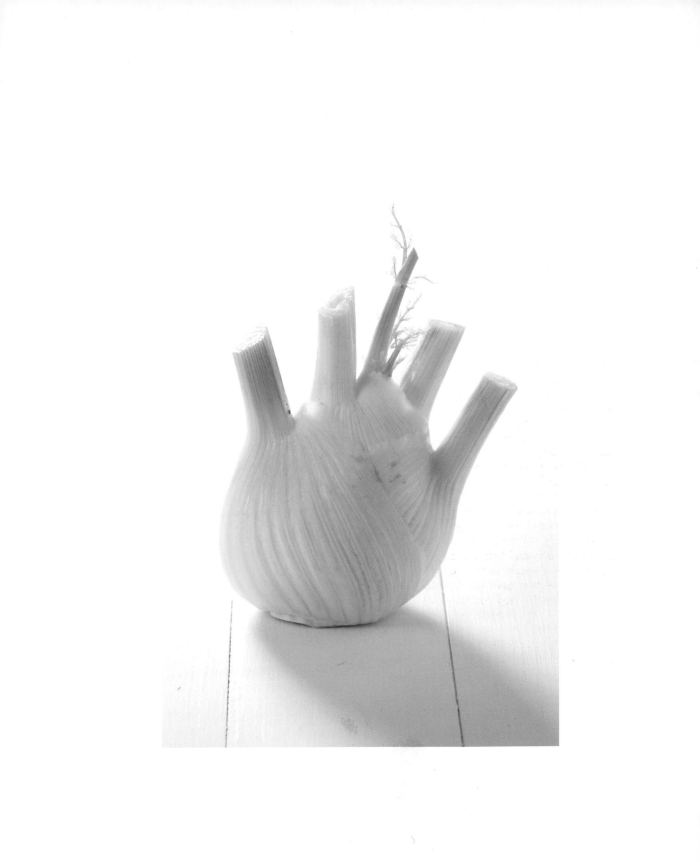

Before you start the 10lb Diet, you will need to analyse your lifestyle. Look at where your lifestyle is right now! Consider the following factors and ask yourself how they have affected your weight.

ALCOHOL

It is very clear that alcohol can cause serious health problems, and we must also look at alcohol from a weightloss point of view. Consider this: 1g alcohol contains 7 kcal. This is second only to fat, which contains 9 kcal/g. Protein and carbohydrates contain only 4 kcal/g. Put these facts into practice and you will find that one small bottle of wine (187ml) has about 20g alcohol. The alcohol alone amounts to 140 kcal. When you add in the sugar and other contents, the calories shoot up even more. And there is little nutritional value: drinking alcohol is simply drinking calories!

Even if we are happy to drink the calories, we must think about the other effects of alcohol. Too much alcohol leads to dehydration and other horrible side effects – it is also the quickest way to derail your diet! I love white wine – Sauvignon Blanc, preferably South African. (Don't forget I lived there for almost five years!) My favourite bottle has just under 10 units of alcohol in it. Shocking, I know! When I talk about units and healthy limits of alcohol with my patients, they are shocked too! We used to say that 14 units a week is a healthy limit for a woman and 21 for a man – but that has changed with new emerging research showing how alcohol is a poison. I get goose bumps (*kananliha* in Finnish) when I say this.

SMOKING

Smoking is the single greatest avoidable risk factor for cancer, and if it is added to the risk of carrying extra weight, you are going to be facing the consequences – guaranteed! I can always smell a smoker and I can also spot them in a crowd: lines around the lips, and damaged skin, hair and teeth. I feel so sorry for smokers and their loved ones. Not only are smokers wasting money but they are also stealing years from their lives.

Whatever about alcohol, there is nothing positive about smoking! All of the research agrees that nicotine and other chemicals in cigarettes will reduce the absorption of vital nutrients and will weaken your immune system. I don't want to send you on a guilt trip, but smoking is a drastic threat to your health – and drastic measures are required!

This is a weightloss book. However, if you are a smoker, I am asking you to address that issue first. Stop smoking! If you want to change your life, your appearance and your health … you can. You can do the weightloss plan and stop smoking all in one go. If there is a will, there is a way. You will thank me in the end. And your loved ones will be happy that I am being tough on you. Sometimes you need to be unkind in order to be kind. There is nothing cool or sexy about smoking!

DIABETES

So many people suffer from prediabetes that I have adopted the following opinion in my clinics: *everybody suffers from diabetes, unless it can be proven otherwise!* Type 2 diabetes (T2DM) has reached such a worldwide epidemic that this opinion does not feel like an exaggeration to me. The worst thing is that the primary cause for 90% of T2DM is actually *obesity*. This means that the disease is preventable! Why is it that we turn to drugs for this problem, when we should look at weightloss first?

If we reduce carbohydrates and calories in the diet, we will force the body to utilise its own stores of energy. This will bring weightloss, improved glucose levels, improved insulin sensitivity and, most important, lowered levels of produced insulin. Sensible weightloss can achieve all of these things and help to prevent major health problems further down the line.

SLEEP DISORDERS

Sleep helps our bodies to regenerate. Most of us need an average of 8 hours of sleep per night (me included). However, we know that 1 in 10 people suffer from insomnia and 3 in 10 feel sleep-deprived. How is this linked to weightloss?

Sleep disturbance is a sign that something is wrong: in order to sleep well, you need to *be* well! Lifestyle choices (e.g. caffeine, alcohol and lack of exercise) affect the quality of our sleep. When I ask my patients how excess weight has affected them, without fail they will say 'low energy levels'. Of course, carrying excess weight is physically tiring – but there is more to the low energy levels. Low energy levels are really bad news for your health: they lead to poor motivation and bad choices. We have a saying in my native Finland: *Sleeping is like putting money in the bank.* Take some good advice from Finland. Mind your sleep and you will be better able to take care of your weight also!

Once you have analysed your lifestyle, you know where things are *now*. The next step is motivation: thinking about where you *want* to be! Motivation is all about clear goals – and 10lb is a very clear goal.

Once you set this goal for yourself, you can decide whether it is something you will do by yourself or with a partner or friend.

I believe that the reason many people postpone their goals is seldom down to laziness, but rather the fear of not succeeding. Don't let this happen to you! Set a clear goal, commit to 10lb and really go for it.

It helps if you have a clear plan. Try to visualise your goal. What do you want at the end of the process? Do you want to be a size 12 again? Do you want to reduce the effects of your diabetes? Do you want a six-pack? Whatever it is, write it down on paper and be descriptive! This will be your motivation to keep going if things get tough. You must remember where it is you want to go!

COMMIT TO THE RULES

You can read more about the Fast Plan and the Slow Plan from p.10 onwards. But whether you choose the Fast Plan or the Slow Plan, there are certain lifestyle rules that should always apply. I like the number 13: for me, this is a list to live by!

1 Sleep well

2 Eat regularly

3 Plan your meals

4 When you are eating, focus on eating

5 Be active every day

6 Eat protein with every meal

7 Eat fruit or vegetables with every meal

8 Get your daily intake of unsaturated fats

9 Drink 2 litres of liquids every day

10 Eat real, unprocessed food

11 Consume fish oil, magnesium and Vitamin D3 every day

12 Don't forget the final touch: make an effort with your hair, clothes and makeup

13 Follow these rules 80% of the time – and forgive yourself for the other 20%.

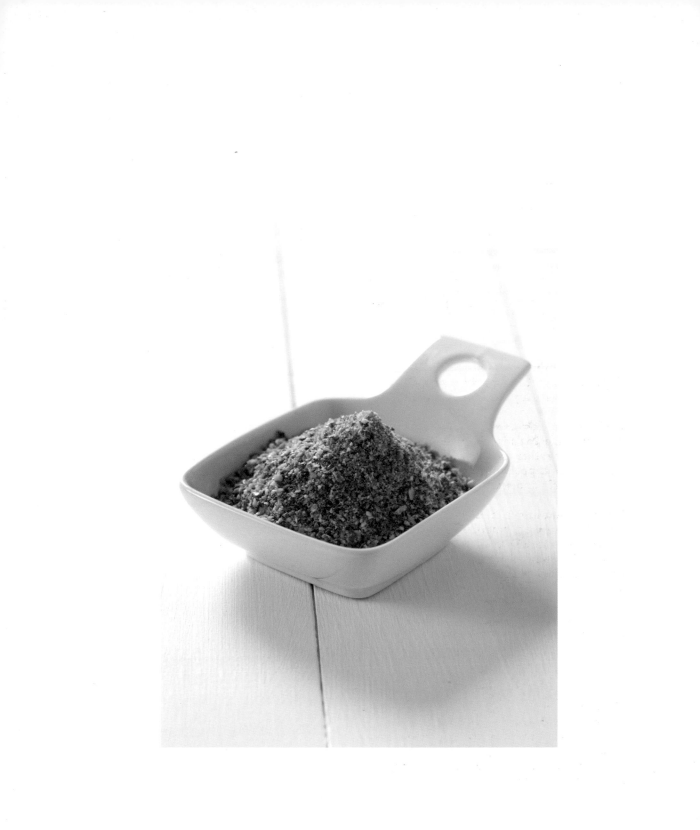

It is difficult to quantify exactly how many calories a person needs in a day.

It depends on so many variables (age, gender, medication, exercise levels, previous diet history, etc.) that I could write a whole chapter on the subject. The official guidelines say that the average woman needs 2000 kcal per day to maintain her weight – and the average man needs 2500 kcal. In reality, this doesn't seem to be the case for the average person that I see in my clinic.

The 10lb Diet is built on my belief that the average woman needs around 1800 kcal per day to maintain her weight. The average man needs around 2200 kcal per day. But if these are the amounts for maintaining weight, what can we do when we want to *lose* weight?

People say that weightloss is difficult – but in many ways it is very simple. Use more energy than you take in, and you will lose weight! We have seen the health improvements that can come from losing 10lb. Of course, there are many different ways to get to that goal. Here, I offer you two different plans. It is up to you to choose what will work for you. As I always say: 'All roads lead to Rome!'

FAST PLAN

Lose 10lb in 3 WEEKS

1000 kcal per day

Eat breakfast, lunch and dinner

Snack carefully throughout the week

Avoid alcohol

Exercise: burn 200 kcal per day

SLOW PLAN

Lose 10lb in 12 WEEKS

1300 kcal per day

Eat breakfast, lunch and dinner

Snack moderately throughout the week

Enjoy alcohol in moderation

Exercise: burn 200 kcal per day

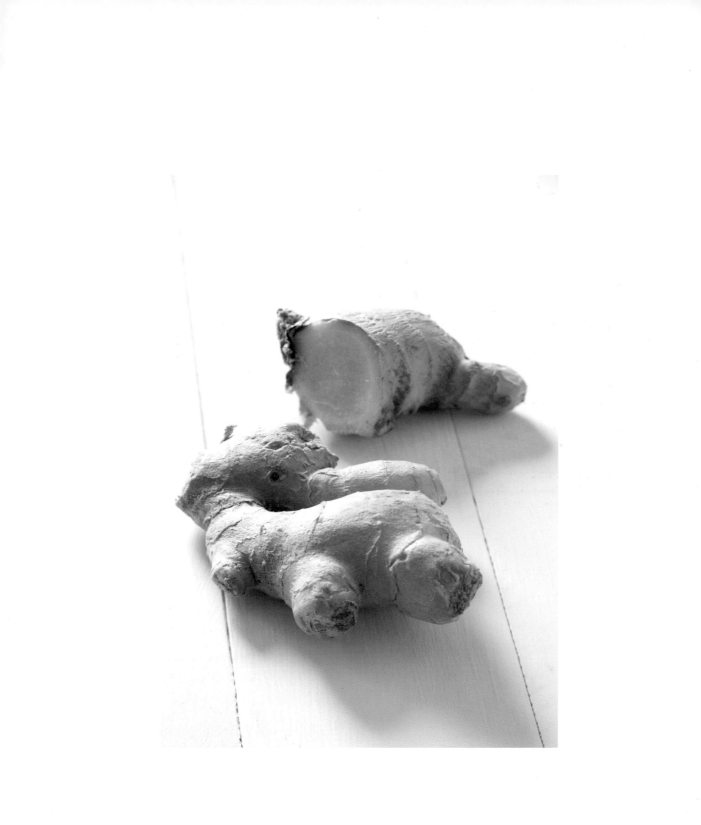

If you can identify with any of these statements, consider doing the Fast Plan.

- I am totally fed up trying to lose just 10lb of weight – I just want to see results immediately!

- I have gone through a major change in life (e.g. having a baby) and I have gained 10lb really quickly. Now I want to lose it quickly.

- I am just back from the holiday of a lifetime – but I am 10lb heavier than when I left...

- I am facing a medical procedure and I need to get in shape really quickly.

- I need to lose more than 10lb but I know I won't continue with my weightloss journey unless I get off to a brilliant start.

- My GP tells me that my cholesterol/blood sugar level is not healthy. If I lose some weight, maybe I won't need to go on medication.

- I have lost a lot of weight but I cannot seem to shift the final 10lb: they are just so stubborn!

HOW DOES THE FAST PLAN WORK?

On the Fast Plan, you restrict your calorie intake to 1000 kcal per day and create a further daily energy deficit of 200 kcal through exercise.

You need to stick to 1000 kcal per day, so it's all about planning! Get a pen and paper and plan your meals to suit your day. Take a look at my sample Diet Diaries on pp.24–26 but remember you can mix and match. Try out new recipes and meal options – and adapt the plans to suit *you*.

So, if Monday morning is mayhem in your house (as it is in mine), don't take on the Courgette and Bacon Pancake! Have 'breakfast on the go' with the Raspberry Smoothie. If Sunday is a quiet day for you, the Seafood Rice Paper Rolls would be perfect for lunch. If you have a craving for a curry on Saturday night, try making the Chicken Tikka Masala. You get the picture!

TIPS FOR THE FAST PLAN

It can be difficult to stay within the 1000 kcal daily limit for 3 weeks. Here are some tips for you.

- Think of your day as three targets:
  - ☐ 200 kcal for breakfast + morning snack
  - ☐ 300 kcal for lunch + afternoon snack
  - ☐ 500 kcal for dinner + evening snack.

- Snacks are vital in the first week of the Fast Plan, especially since you might be used to snacking a lot. Plan them carefully, though!

- Eat Filler Soups – see pp.64–79. They are a smart way to keep the hunger pangs at bay while you stay within your calorie limit.

- Avoid alcohol: it will make you too hungry and too relaxed. You might forget that you are on the Fast Plan!

- Vary your recipes and meal options so that your diet is interesting and nutritious.

- Remember: you don't have to cook every single meal. Create a weekly plan that includes recipes and meal options that are readily available.

If you can identify with any of these statements, consider doing the Slow Plan.

- I don't want to make a radical change to my diet but I do want a lifestyle change, with better food choices.

- I have gained 10lb over the years. I don't need to lose it overnight, but I do want to lose it.

- I want to 'clean up my act' but I still want to be able to eat out and have a drink or two.

- My clothes feel a bit tight recently. I want to shed 10lb to feel really comfortable again.

- I want to lose 10lb but I don't want the whole world to know about it! I'd rather not talk about it with family or friends. I just want to lose 10lb and feel the difference.

- I have been through some health issues recently. While I recover, I want to slowly lose a bit of weight to improve my overall health.

- I did the Fast Plan – I lost 10lb and I feel fantastic! Now I want to take things easier and lose the next 10lb a bit more slowly.

HOW DOES THE SLOW PLAN WORK?

On the Slow Plan, you restrict your calorie intake to 1300 kcal per day and create a further daily energy deficit of 200 kcal through exercise.

You are aiming for 1300 kcal per day. You don't need to stick too rigidly to this, but you still must plan your meals to suit your lifestyle. Take a look at my sample Diet Diaries on pp.27–29. Remember that you have plenty of time on the Slow Plan, so try out lots of different recipes and meal options. Once you stick to the 1300 kcal limit overall, you can adapt the plan to suit *you*.

So, if you like baking, the Granola Protein Bars would be a useful breakfast option. You can have them wrapped in the fridge and ready to go. If it's winter and you feel like a hearty lunch, then make the Potato and Leek Soup. If it's summer and you feel like having a barbecue with some friends, make the Chicken Kebabs for dinner. You can even enjoy a drink or two!

TIPS FOR THE SLOW PLAN

The Slow Plan is not too strict but you must still meet your target over 12 weeks, so stay on track! Here are some tips for you.

■ Think of your day as two targets:
   □ 600 kcal for breakfast + morning snack + lunch
   □ 700 kcal for afternoon snack + dinner + evening snack.

■ Every daily choice matters, but do not worry if you cannot stick to your exact plan for the day. The goal is to stick to the 1300 kcal limit and to get your daily exercise.

■ Focus on changing your eating habits. The Slow Plan is not about speed: make an effort to change your lifestyle!

■ Think about what you will eat in the 12 weeks ahead. Make recipes that freeze well. This is crucial: otherwise, you will fall back into old habits and forget about the fact that you are trying to lose weight!

■ Since you have just two targets in the day, think about how to space out your calories. Eat when you are hungry and stop when you are full.

■ I don't need to lecture you about alcohol and the infamous 'empty calories' it brings. You can enjoy alcohol sensibly on the Slow Plan. And if you don't want to drink, help yourself to some extra snacks instead.

> Whichever plan you choose, you must aim for nutritional balance, regular exercise and healthy lifestyle choices. Listen to your body – and to your GP!

EXERCISE PLAN

HOW MUCH EXERCISE DO I NEED?

Whether you are on the Fast Plan or the Slow Plan, you must aim to burn 200 kcal per day through exercise. Your daily exercise can be split into two parts:

- 10 minutes of cardiovascular exercise
- 10 minutes of weight/core training.

This should give you a calorie deficit of 150–200 kcal daily. Obviously, a lot depends on your starting weight, fitness levels and mobility. Try to challenge yourself and push yourself out of the 'comfort zone' whenever you can!

It is vital that you make the time to exercise every day. If you cannot manage a 20-minute exercise session in one go, split it up throughout the day. Here are some examples that my patients have tried in the past.

Monday
- 10 minutes: dancing (high intensity!)
- 10 minutes: weight/core training

Tuesday
- 10 minutes: Nordic walking
- 10 minutes: weight/core training

Wednesday
- 20 minutes: swimming (total body workout, so weight/core training is not needed here)

Thursday
- 10 minutes: dancing
- 10 minutes: weight/core training

Friday
- 10 minutes: aerobics exercises
- 10 minutes: weight/core training

Saturday
- 10 minutes: Nordic walking
- 10 minutes: weight/core training

Sunday
- 20 minutes: swimming

TIPS FOR THE EXERCISE PLAN

- I suggest cardiovascular exercise first thing in the morning. If you do it in the morning, then it is out of the way and you don't have to worry about motivational levels later on in the day.

- Even when you are not 'exercising' you have the opportunity to keep your body moving. Sometimes exercise does not necessarily look like exercise: when you are lifting boxes at work or playing with your children, you might actually call this weight training! To have a more targeted approach to your fitness routine, however, I recommend you do the specific exercises in this book.

- In order to be successful on the 10lb Diet, you must prioritise *yourself*. If this means that your family or your work do not get your undivided attention for 100% of the day, don't feel guilty. Do your best every day and remember that it is only when you take care of your health that you can take care of other things too.

- The warm-up is a vital part of any workout. A good warm-up will ensure that you gradually increase your heart rate to the required level and mobilise your muscles and joints.

- Cardiovascular exercise should make you feel warm and sweaty. If you are not sweating, then you are not doing enough!

- You must start and finish each weight/core training session with some gentle stretches in order to avoid injury.

- Some people worry that weight/core training will create huge muscles – it won't! Basic weight/core training will simply result in a more toned figure.

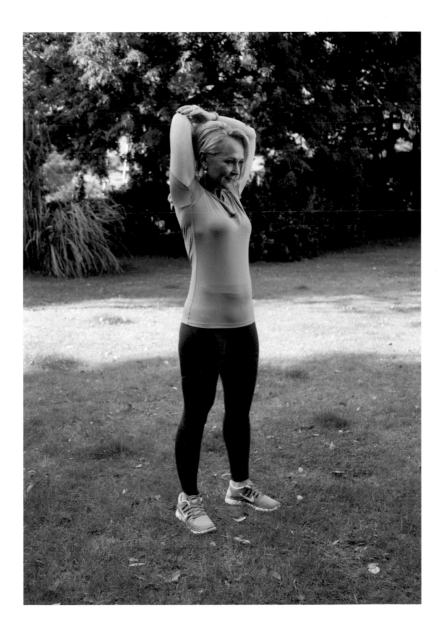

In my view, these six exercises are essential for daily health.

EXERCISE 1: ONE-ARM DUMBBELL ROW

- Complete 3 sets of 10/15 repetitions
- 4kg dumbbell

Start with your left knee and left hand on a bench, while your right leg is planted on the ground. Bend forward and point your hip bones straight down and make sure your torso is parallel to the ground. Do not shrug your shoulders up and down: keep them fixed, bringing the dumbbell up close to the body while flexing the elbow only. Exhale on the effort. This exercise can also be done on the floor.

EXERCISE 2: LATERAL AND FRONT RAISE (COMBINED)

- Complete 3 sets of 10/15 repetitions
- 3kg dumbbells for first set
- 2kg dumbbells for second and third sets

Hold a set of 3kg dumbbells for your first set. Begin with a side raise, lifting the dumbbells out from the sides of your body up to shoulder height. Return to starting position and then complete a front raise with palms facing down and hands straight in front of the body, just to shoulder height. Keep abdominals engaged and avoid swinging your back. After the first set, drop to 2kg dumbbells to complete the workout. Exhale on the effort, as your arms come up.

EXERCISE 3: BICEP CURLS

- Complete 3 sets of 10/15 repetitions
- 3kg dumbbells

Hold the dumbbells, palms facing up, keeping the elbows tucked in close to your body. Exhale and bend the elbows all the way up, return down in a slow and controlled movement.

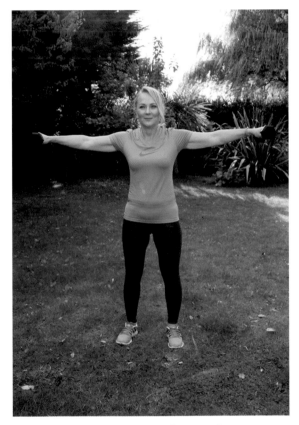

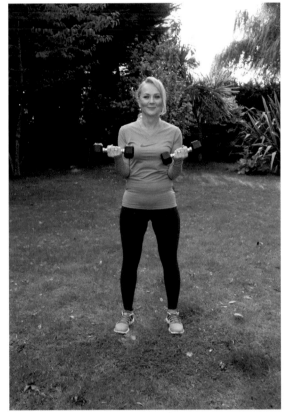

Exercise 2: Lateral and front raise (combined)

Exercise 3: Bicep curls

EXERCISE 4: ABDOMINAL CURL

- Complete 2 sets of 10/15 repetitions

Lie on your back, with knees bent at 45 degrees and feet flat on the floor. Place your hands beside your head, elbows pointing out and chin slightly lifted towards the ceiling. As you lift your back off the mat, exhale on the effort. Avoid pulling your head with your hands.

EXERCISE 5: LUNGES

- Complete 3 sets of 10/15 repetitions
- 3kg dumbbells

Hold the dumbbells at the sides of your body. Start with your feet together and take a large step forward; once your front heel hits the ground, lower your hips to the ground until both knees are bent. Return to the starting position. Repeat. Keep abdominals engaged and spine straight. Do not let your front knee pass your toes.

EXERCISE 6: SIT/STAND OFF THE CHAIR

- Complete 3 sets of 10/15 repetitions

Find a comfortable and stable chair. Repeat the movement of sitting down on the chair and standing upright. Engage your abdominal muscles both when sitting and standing up. To make it harder, try not to use your hands.

NORDIC WALKING

Nordic walking is a simple exercise that gives serious results! You can buy Nordic walking poles in any good outdoors/sports shop. Many people cannot jog or run because of the strain on their knees or because of other mobility issues. With Nordic walking, the physical strain is evenly distributed throughout the body, so there is little risk of injury. It is a great way to burn calories and increase aerobic fitness – and it is fun too!

KEGEL EXERCISES are essential for women, since these exercises strengthen the pelvic floor muscles. Performing a Kegel is an internal movement, with no external muscle involvement. It can be performed anywhere and at any time with no extra equipment. To understand the movement involved in performing a Kegel, imagine you have to urinate but must hold it in until you can get to a bathroom, or imagine trying to stop urination in mid-stream. Repeat Kegel exercises as often as possible: in the car, while watching TV, or before falling asleep at night.

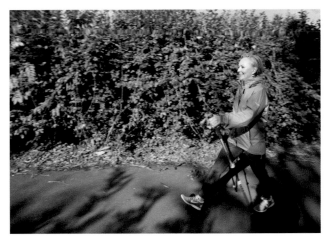

Nordic walking

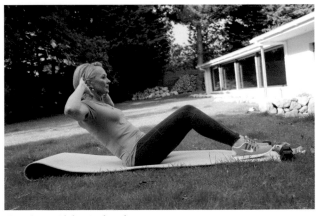

Exercise 4: Abdominal curl

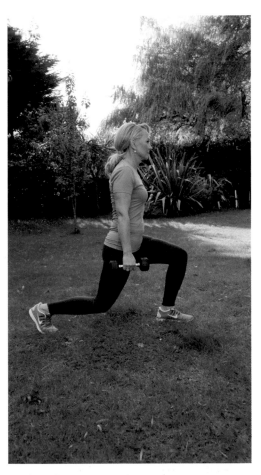

Exercise 5: Lunges

I created the 10lb Diet by following the same principle we follow in my clinics. People find it easier to stick to a plan that is already made rather than trying to choose from a list of 'allowed' items or 'points'! Our type of meal planning helps you in your shopping, since you can clearly see what you need for the week ahead.

The Diet Diaries on pp.24–29 are examples only, so feel free to change them to suit your taste and lifestyle. To help keep it simple, you can bulk prepare and freeze plenty of the meals.

The sample Diet Diaries give you a general idea of the calories of some standard ingredients. Remember that fruit and vegetable sizes vary, so keep an eye on your portions. Also remember that calories are very different between brands of foods, so one brand of rye cracker is likely to be different from another!

The 10lb Diet offers you plenty to eat. It just takes a bit of organisation to plan your meals. You will see that this is not just some 'eat less' plan. If you prepare properly, it is an interesting, fresh and varied diet!

Whether you are on the Fast Plan or the Slow Plan, use the template below to plan your meals and snacks. You can download the blank template at www.gillmacmillanbooks.ie.

To help you get started, I've written three sample weeks for the Fast Plan (pp.24–26) and three sample weeks for the Slow Plan (pp.27–29). It is important that you adapt the plans to suit your lifestyle.

	SUNDAY	MONDAY	TUESDAY	WEDNESDAY	THURSDAY	FRIDAY	SATURDAY
BREAKFAST							
MORNING SNACK							
LUNCH							
AFTERNOON SNACK							
DINNER							
EVENING SNACK							
DAILY KCAL TOTAL							

FAST PLAN 1000 KCAL WEEK 1

	SUNDAY	MONDAY	TUESDAY	WEDNESDAY	THURSDAY	FRIDAY	SATURDAY
BREAKFAST	Scrambled Eggs with Caviar (168)	35g muesli with 150ml low fat milk (194)	Porridge (40g oats) made with water (156)	Raspberry Smoothie (195)	Buckwheat Flatbread with 5g butter (138)	Finnish Whipped Porridge with 100ml low fat milk (189)	1 Weetabix with 150ml low fat natural yoghurt and 100g blueberries (196)
MORNING SNACK	Hot Chocolate (84)	Cappuccino made with 100ml light soya milk (22)	Small apple (50)	Babybel light cheese (42)	Diet yoghurt with 150g strawberries (95)	Satsuma (40)	
LUNCH	Leek and Potato Soup (238)	Borscht (357)	3 rye crackers, 3 slices of cold meat, light cheese spread and Tomato Soup (279)	Waldorf Salad (258)	Fish Soup (271)	Spinach and Feta Quesadilla with Celeriac Mushroom Soup (175)	3 rye crispbreads, 1 boiled egg and Celeriac Mushroom Soup (221)
AFTERNOON SNACK	Finnish Whipped Porridge (147)	Baba Ganoush with 2 oatcakes (127)	2 ginger oat biscuits (86)	Buckwheat Flatbread with 5g butter (138)	Baba Ganoush, 3 rye crackers and sliced cucumber (151)	5 Brazil nuts (100)	Granola Protein Bar with Hot Chocolate (258)
DINNER	Fried Halloumi with Cumin-Spiced Leeks (359)	Portuguese Squid with Cauliflower Mash (399)	Portion of oily fish with Cauliflower Mash and steamed broccoli (400)	Fish with Mushroom Sauce (368)	Chicken Butternut Bake (347)	Cowboy Stew (475)	Chicken Tikka Masala (327)
EVENING SNACK						Curry dip with red peppers and celery (40)	
DAILY KCAL TOTAL	996 KCAL	1099 KCAL	971 KCAL	1001 KCAL	1002 KCAL	1019 KCAL	1002 KCAL

FAST PLAN 1000 KCAL WEEK 2

	SUNDAY	MONDAY	TUESDAY	WEDNESDAY	THURSDAY	FRIDAY	SATURDAY
BREAKFAST	Porridge (40g oats) made with 200ml low fat milk (240)	2 grilled bacon medallions, 1 poached egg and 100g steamed mushrooms (136)	Granola Protein Bar (174)	Dr Eva's Eggs Benedict (266)	1 boiled egg, 1 slice of wholemeal soda bread and 5g butter (190)	45g muesli with 200ml light soya milk (212)	Barley Porridge (315)
MORNING SNACK	Satsuma (40)	Small apple (50)	3 thin rice cakes, 2 light cheese spreads (107)	125ml natural yoghurt with 100g strawberries (112)			
LUNCH	Warm Halloumi Salad and Tomato Soup (293)	Pork Sausage Soup (306)	Wholemeal pitta with 80g cooked chicken and 15ml extra light mayo, and Pea and Mint Soup (260)	Wholemeal wrap with Creamy Salmon Pâté and iceberg lettuce, and Pea and Mint Soup (188)	Russian Soup (319)	2 slices of Ultimate Health Loaf, 10g butter, and Creamy Chorizo Soup (272)	Dill-cured Salmon Tartare (381)
AFTERNOON SNACK		Courgette hummus with cucumber sticks (50)					
DINNER	Stuffed Onions (419)	Spicy Chicken Tacos (447)	Prawn Stir-Fry (310)	Vegetable Fajitas (422)	Easy Fish Pie (549)	Russian Soup (319)	Turkey Burgers with Celeriac Chips (315)
EVENING SNACK			100g low fat cottage cheese and 100g tinned peaches in juice (135)			Coconut Biscuit with 200ml low fat milk (210)	
DAILY KCAL TOTAL	992 KCAL	989 KCAL	986 KCAL	988 KCAL	1058 KCAL	1013 KCAL	1011 KCAL

FAST PLAN 1000 KCAL WEEK 3

	SUNDAY	MONDAY	TUESDAY	WEDNESDAY	THURSDAY	FRIDAY	SATURDAY
BREAKFAST	2 Buckwheat Flatbreads with light cheese spread (255)	Banana Pancake with 100g blueberries (201)	100g baked beans and 1 small slice brown bread (141)	45g Shredded Wheat with 150ml low fat milk (248)	Barley Porridge (315)	Skagen (296)	Courgette and Bacon Pancake (152)
MORNING SNACK	Miso soup (29)	Kiwi (69)	Dark chocolate bar (85%) with Hot Chocolate (229)				125ml natural yoghurt (82)
LUNCH	Bacon and Halloumi Stew (186)	1 large slice of rye bread, 2 slices of cold turkey and Celery and Roquefort Soup (225)	Sushi Salad (255)	Carvery lunch: 1 slice of turkey breast, 1 portion of steamed carrots and 1 scoop of mash (385)	McDonald's hamburger (250)	Wholemeal wrap with Mackerel Pâté and Tricolour Soup (174)	Tex-Mex Salad (488)
AFTERNOON SNACK	Small tub of low fat hummus with carrot sticks (190)	125ml natural yogurt with 100g raspberries (112)	Boiled egg (70)	Small apple (50)	Tricolour Soup (88)	Satsuma (40)	Kiwi (69)
DINNER	2-egg omelette with peppers, mushrooms and scallion, and steamed French beans (180)	Chilli Pasta Bolognese (378)	Creamy Prawn Risotto (310)	Borscht (357)	Creamy Ham and Garlic Pasta (365)	Meal out: Grilled white fish, green side salad and steamed broccoli and asparagus (350)	Vegetable Green Curry (172)
EVENING SNACK	Granola Protein Bar (174)					2 oatcakes with light cheese spread (141)	Celery sticks with horseradish and herb dip (32)
DAILY KCAL TOTAL	1014 KCAL	985 KCAL	1005 KCAL	1040 KCAL	1018 KCAL	1001 KCAL	995 KCAL

SLOW PLAN 1300 KCAL WEEK 1

	SUNDAY	MONDAY	TUESDAY	WEDNESDAY	THURSDAY	FRIDAY	SATURDAY
BREAKFAST	Granola Protein Bar (174)	Barley Porridge (315)	100g baked beans and 1 slice of wholemeal soda bread (174)	Banana Pancake (171)	2 Weetabix with 200ml low fat natural yoghurt (266)	Purple 'Pick Me Up' Juice (143)	Dr Eva's Eggs Benedict (266)
MORNING SNACK			Light Soya Latte made with 200ml light soya milk (44)	Kiwi (69)		Medium avocado (280)	
LUNCH	Russian Soup with 1 slice of wholemeal soda bread and 5g butter (439)	Russian Soup (319)	Two wholemeal wraps with 1 large tin of salmon and 30ml extra light mayo, and Tricolour Soup (396)	Turkish Pizza (570)	Potato and Leek Soup with 1 slice of wholemeal soda bread (324)	Baked potato (200g) with 2 portions of Creamy Salmon Pâté, and High Fibre Salad (304)	4 rye crackers with 4 slices of turkey and 2 portions of low fat cheese, and Tom Yum soup (383)
AFTERNOON SNACK	2 plums (60)						
DINNER	Chicken Kebabs with Pomegranate Molasses and 50g brown basmati rice (uncooked weight) (411)	Chicken Fried Rice (481) (using leftover rice from night before)	Farmer's Pie (515)	Fish Rolls with Cauliflower Mash (338)	Easy Fish Pie (549)	Meal out: 180g fillet steak with steamed vegetables (380)	Vegetarian Sausage Stew (447)
EVENING SNACK	2 measures of vodka with 1 Diet Coke (160)	Granola Protein Bar (174)	Great Grandma's Berry Soup with 100ml low fat milk (189)	Great Grandma's Berry Soup (147)	3 oatcakes with Creamy Salmon Pâté (159)	2 x 187ml glasses of red wine (254)	White Wine Sangria (221)
DAILY KCAL TOTAL	1244 KCAL	1289 KCAL	1318 KCAL	1295 KCAL	1298 KCAL	1361 KCAL	1317 KCAL

SLOW PLAN 1300 KCAL WEEK 2

	SUNDAY	MONDAY	TUESDAY	WEDNESDAY	THURSDAY	FRIDAY	SATURDAY
BREAKFAST	Courgette and Bacon Pancake (152)	Raspberry Smoothie (195)	Porridge (40g oats) made with 200ml low fat milk (240)	2 Oatibix with 200ml low fat milk (294)	Scrambled Eggs with Caviar and 1 large slice of rye bread (300)	2 Buckwheat Flatbreads and 10g butter (274)	Grill: 2 bacon medallions, 1 turkey sausage, 1 poached egg, 1 slice of wholemeal soda bread, 5g butter and 100g baked beans (400)
MORNING SNACK	3 rye crackers, 1 portion of soft cheese and sliced cucumber (154)	Coconut Biscuit (126)	Boiled egg (70)	100g Greek yoghurt with 100g strawberries (160)	200g Greek yogurt with 30g blueberries (290)	3 plums (90)	3 Brazil nuts (60)
LUNCH	Borscht (357)	Pork Sausage Soup (306)	4 rye crackers, 4 slices of ham, 10g butter and Pea and Mint Soup (346)	Wholemeal wrap with 80g cooked chicken and 15ml extra light mayo, and Pea and Mint Soup (260)	Borscht with 1 large slice of rye bread and 5g butter (402)	Chilli Pasta Bolognese (378)	Warm Halloumi Salad (196)
AFTERNOON SNACK	Granola Protein Bar (174)	Kiwi (69)	Latte made with 200ml low fat milk (84)			Coconut Biscuit (126)	Ryvita minis (90)
DINNER	Easy Cauliflower Carbonara (538)	Lamb Rogan Josh (548)	Yellow Dal (532)	Spicy Chicken Tacos and 1 light beer (547)	Fish with Mushroom Sauce (368)	Portuguese Squid with Cauliflower Mash (399)	Meal out: 180g fillet of salmon, side salad and steamed vegetables (420)
EVENING SNACK		Babybel light (42)					187ml glass of white wine (145)
DAILY KCAL TOTAL	1375 KCAL	1286 KCAL	1272 KCAL	1261 KCAL	1360 KCAL	1267 KCAL	1311 KCAL

SLOW PLAN 1300 KCAL WEEK 3

	SUNDAY	MONDAY	TUESDAY	WEDNESDAY	THURSDAY	FRIDAY	SATURDAY
BREAKFAST	2 scrambled eggs, 1 large slice of rye bread and 5g butter (308)	Skagen (296)	Finnish Whipped Porridge with 100ml low fat milk (189)	2 Weetabix with 200ml light soya milk (182)	50g granola with 200ml low fat natural yoghurt (352)	Raspberry Smoothie (195)	Barley Porridge with Great Grandma's Berry Soup (462)
MORNING SNACK		2 kiwi (140)	15g bag of popcorn (68)	3 thin rice cakes with Smoked Mackerel Pâté and sliced cucumber (87)			Rooibos and Apple Iced Tea (16)
LUNCH	Carvery lunch: 1 slice of roast beef, 1 portion of steamed carrots and 1 scoop of mash (420)	McDonald's Grilled Chicken Wrap, and Celery Roquefort Soup (291)	Fish Soup with 1 large slice of rye bread, 1 slice of Cheddar and 5g butter (499)	Wholemeal wrap with 3 slices of ham, 1 portion of low fat cheese, and Tomato Soup (264)	Farmer's Pie (515) (leftovers from the day before)	Tex-Mex Salad (488)	Spinach and Feta Quesadilla with Tomato Soup (193)
AFTERNOON SNACK	Dark chocolate bar (85%) with Hot Chocolate (229)	100g low fat cottage cheese with 100g peaches (135)	Granola Protein Bar (174)				5 Brazil nuts and 1 diet yoghurt (150)
DINNER	2 slices of wholemeal soda bread, 2 slices of Cheddar, and Celery Roquefort Soup (343)	Creamy Ham and Garlic Pasta (365)	Chilli Pasta Bolognese (378)	Farmer's Pie (515)	Portuguese squid and 2 medium-sized potatoes (steamed) (439)	Creamy Prawn Risotto and 187ml glass of white wine (465)	Cowboy Stew (475)
EVENING SNACK		2 plums (60)		187ml glass of white wine and Ryvita minis (235)		Finnish Whipped Porridge (147)	
DAILY KCAL TOTAL	1300 KCAL	1287 KCAL	1308 KCAL	1283 KCAL	1306 KCAL	1295 KCAL	1296 KCAL

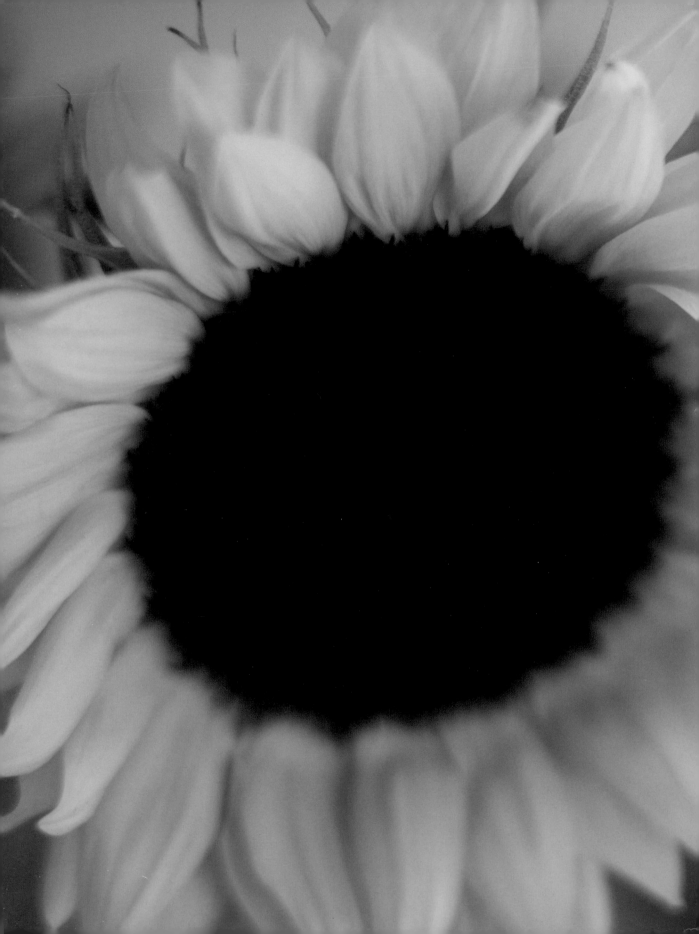

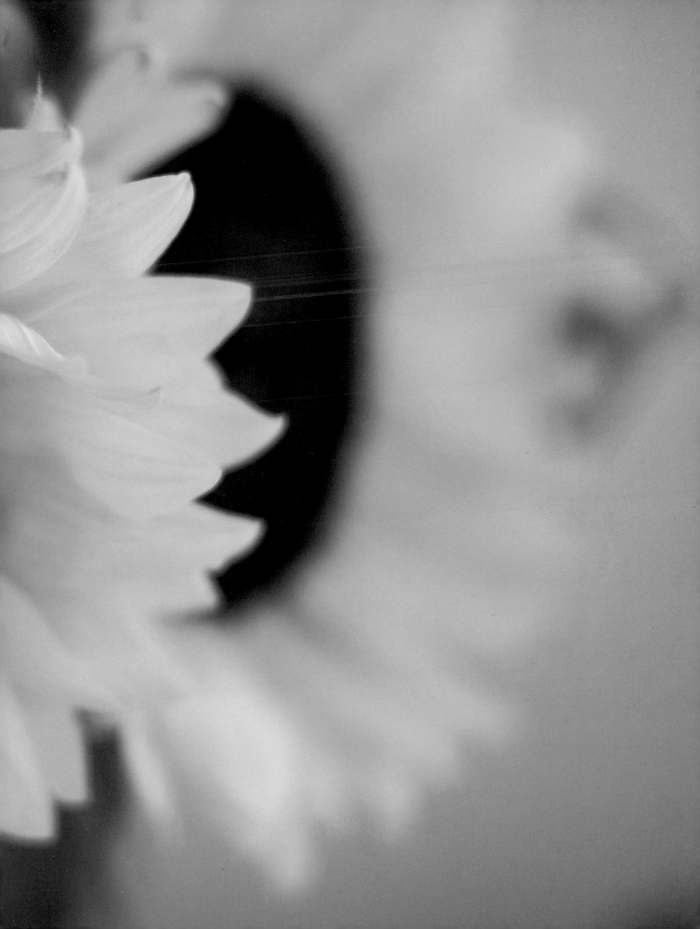

Breakfast

We have been told that breakfast is the most important meal of the day: *Eat breakfast like a king, lunch like a prince and dinner like a pauper.* I don't know if I totally agree with this. Actually, even dogs disagree on this issue: I have two dogs and one of them refuses to eat anything before midday!

The truth is that many people simply do not feel hungry in the morning. So what is the right thing to do? My advice is always to listen to your body. However, I do urge you to eat something for breakfast every day – even if it is light.

Unfortunately, people carrying excess weight often skip breakfast. About 7 out of 10 of my new patients don't want to have breakfast. They tell me: 'I don't feel hungry first thing in the morning.' But then they discover that they are too hungry later on and they reach for a takeaway latte and chocolate muffin on their way to work – it is a total 'carbohydrate time-bomb'! About 700 kcal later, their blood sugars peak and so does their insulin. The result is a massive hunger pang. This could be avoided with a more sensible plan at breakfast time.

I know that everybody's morning routine will be different. Most of us are fighting the clock on weekdays (if you're like me, the clock always seems to win the race), so sitting down to eat a cooked breakfast is a luxury that happens only at the weekends.

This is why the breakfast recipes are varied. Some are substantial and they will carry you through a busy morning of work. Some are light and fresh, so that they feel like a detox if you've overindulged the previous day. Some can be prepared in advance, which means you can eat breakfast and blow-dry your hair at the same time!

Dr Eva's Eggs Benedict

This delicious breakfast will set you up for the day! Having eggs in the morning will keep your hunger pangs at bay. In this recipe, I use 50g ham – but it's equally good with 25g smoked salmon. **Serves 1**

75g spinach leaves, trimmed and washed
1 egg
50g ham, thinly sliced
30g low fat crème fraîche
20g Parmesan, grated
Paprika or cayenne pepper
Salt and pepper

Preheat the grill to medium.

Cook the spinach in a steamer for 3 minutes. Squeeze out the excess water and finely chop the spinach. Set aside and keep warm.

Poach the egg (according to whatever method suits you). Meanwhile, place the cooked spinach on a warmed plate and top with the ham.

As soon as the egg is poached, drain it and place it on top of the ham. Top the egg with the crème fraîche, Parmesan and paprika. Place under the grill until golden brown.

Season and serve without delay.

APPROXIMATELY 266 KCAL, 2.2G FIBRE AND 23.8G PROTEIN PER SERVING

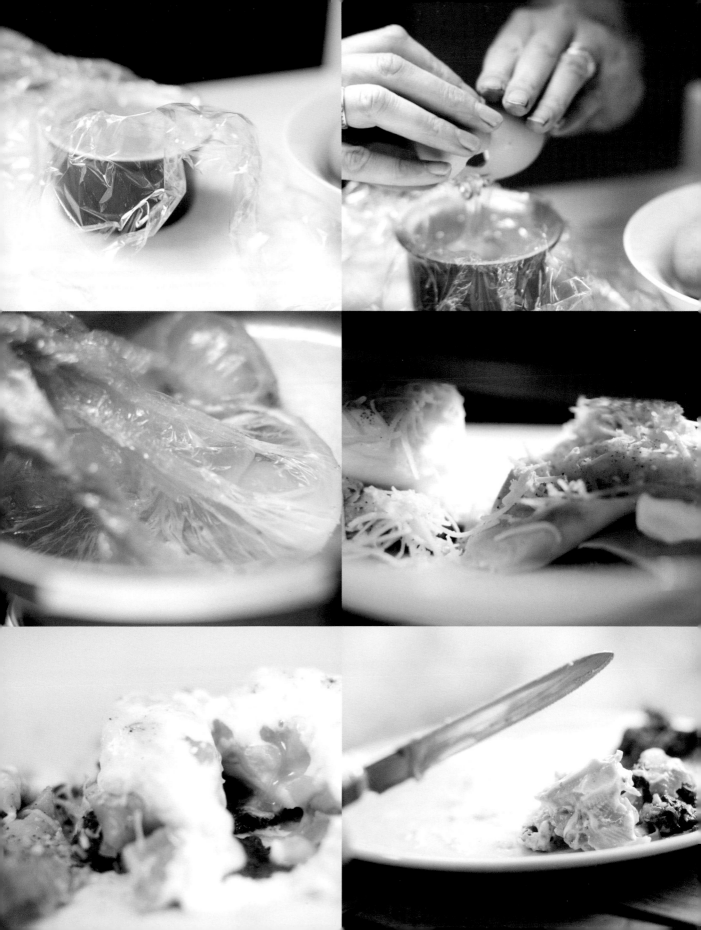

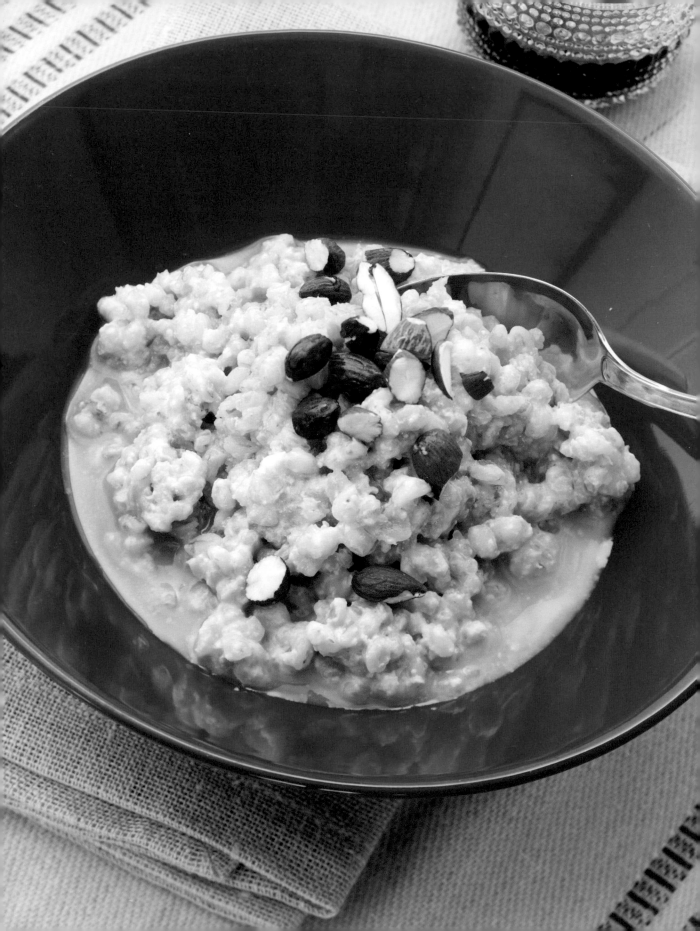

Barley Porridge (Ohraryynipuuro)

Barley has been recognised as a super food since the days of the gladiators! This Barley Porridge is a nice alternative to traditional porridge. The handiest way to cook this recipe is overnight in a slow cooker on a very low setting. Try it with the Kiisseli on p.166. **Serves 4**

200g pearl barley
750ml low fat milk
½ tsp salt
20g butter
Stevia, to serve
20g almonds, to serve (optional)

Place the pearl barley, milk, salt and butter in the slow cooker and set to low. Leave the slow cooker to do the work overnight.

In the morning, give the porridge a stir and serve it with stevia and roughly chopped almonds.

APPROXIMATELY 315 KCAL, 7.8G FIBRE AND 10.6G PROTEIN PER SERVING

Skagen

Skagen is an elegant Swedish speciality of prawns on bread. It was created for the famous Riche restaurant in Stockholm by Tore Wretman in 1958, and it works well for breakfast, brunch or as a snack. I have tweaked the original recipe: my version is low in calories and high in fibre, without any sacrifice on taste. **Serves 4**

400g frozen prawns, thawed, cooked, peeled and chopped
4 tbsp finely chopped fresh dill, plus extra for garnish
1 tbsp mayonnaise
1 tbsp soured cream
1 tbsp Dijon mustard
Juice of ½ lemon
1 tsp horseradish sauce (optional)
12 round crispbreads, such as Finn Crisp (3 per person)
50g herring roe (or caviar!)

Mix the prawns, dill, mayonnaise, soured cream, mustard, lemon juice and horseradish in a medium bowl. Stir well and set aside.

Spread an equal amount of the prawn mixture on each crispbread and top with the herring roe. Garnish with dill and serve.

APPROXIMATELY 296 KCAL, 3.4G FIBRE AND 24.7G PROTEIN PER SERVING

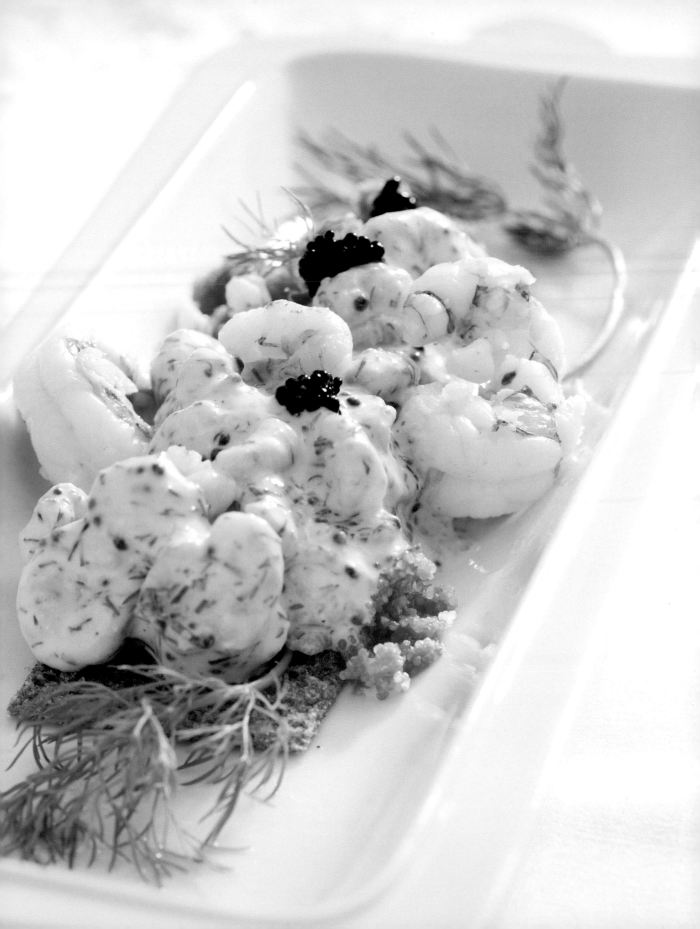

Banana Pancake

This is a wonderful combination of banana and egg. Bananas are such high-energy food and eggs are full of essential amino acids. This pancake can be eaten hot or cold – either way, it's good. **Serves 1**

1 egg
½ a ripe banana, peeled and mashed well
1 tsp butter or 2 tsp coconut oil, for
  frying

Use a whisk to lightly beat the egg in a medium bowl. Add the mashed banana, mix well and set aside.

Heat a non-stick frying pan. Once hot, add the butter and pour in the banana batter, swirling to cover the bottom of the pan. Cook over a low heat for 3 minutes on each side, then slide the pancake onto a warmed serving plate.

APPROXIMATELY 171 KCAL, 1.4G FIBRE AND 7.0G PROTEIN PER SERVING

Courgette and Bacon Pancake

We all love eggs and bacon for breakfast, but this recipe is a healthier and higher fibre alternative to a typical cooked breakfast. If you like, you can use a muffin tin to make individual pancakes that are perfect for breakfast on the go.

I use liquid egg whites from a carton in this recipe – you can find them in most supermarkets. If you don't have Cheddar slices, experiment with a different hard cheese – but make sure to keep the total amount to 240kcal or less! **Serves 4**

250ml egg whites (5 large egg whites)
50ml low fat milk
½ tsp Herbamare herbal salt
Butter
140g bacon medallions, thinly sliced
4 courgettes, finely chopped
1 leek, finely chopped
1 red pepper, finely chopped
4 low fat Cheddar slices

Preheat the oven to 160°C/325°F/gas 3.

Lightly whisk the egg whites, milk and herbal salt in a large bowl and set aside.

Heat 1 teaspoon of butter in a non-stick frying pan. Add the bacon and vegetables and fry for 3–5 minutes.

Place 2 teaspoons of butter in a 41 cm x 24 cm (16 inch x 9 inch) roasting tin and put it in the oven to melt. When the butter has just melted, tip the cooked bacon and vegetables into the roasting tin. Now pour the egg white mixture into the roasting tin, stirring gently.

Return the tin to the oven and cook for 10 minutes. Then add the cheese slices and cook for a further 2–3 minutes. Divide the pancake between warmed serving plates.

APPROXIMATELY 152 KCAL, 2.8G FIBRE AND 15.2G PROTEIN PER SERVING

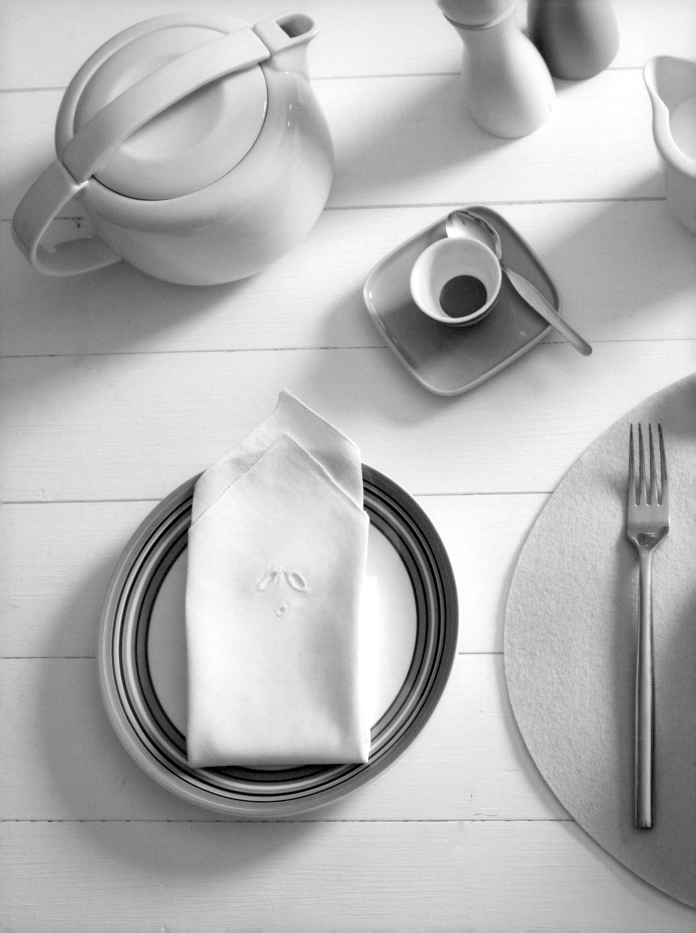

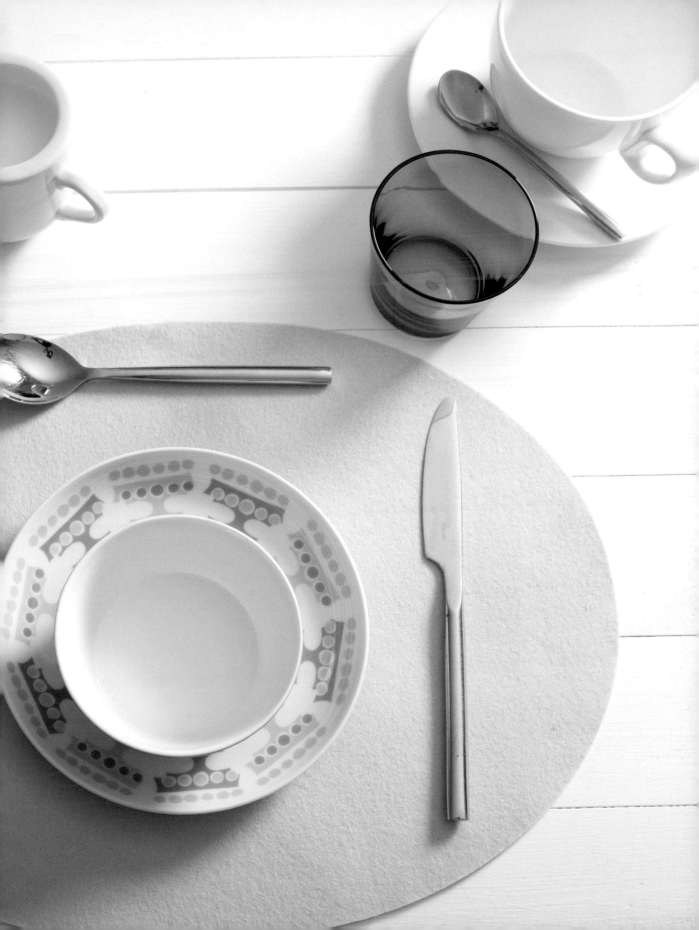

Cauliflower Scrambled Eggs

My two sons love this breakfast – it really fills them up for the day ahead! This recipe is loaded with protein and it has plenty of fibre, so it should help anyone struggling with blood sugar imbalances.

It is a good idea to make the Cauliflower Mash in advance. I make big batches and freeze them. If you defrost the Cauliflower Mash overnight, this becomes a speedy recipe. I don't have much time to spare in the mornings, and I prefer to use my time to do my daily exercises! **Serves 2**

4 eggs, separated into 4 whites and 2 yolks (Use the remaining 2 yolks to make the Mayonnaise on p.196)
2 tbsp low fat soured cream
1 quantity of the Cauliflower Mash on p.184
2 tbsp Parmesan, grated
¼ tsp salt
1 tsp butter
1–2 garlic cloves, crushed (optional)
Freshly ground black pepper
1 tbsp finely chopped fresh herbs (basil, parsley and chives are nice)

Use a whisk to lightly beat the 4 egg whites, 2 egg yolks, soured cream, Cauliflower Mash, Parmesan and salt in a large bowl.

Melt the butter in a large heavy saucepan and pour in the egg mixture. Cook on a low heat for 3–4 minutes, stirring frequently, until the eggs are scrambled but still nice and moist. Stir in the garlic, season and remove from the heat.

Spoon the eggs onto two warmed serving plates and garnish with the chopped herbs.

APPROXIMATELY 310 KCAL, 7.7G FIBRE AND 28.5G PROTEIN PER SERVING

Buckwheat Flatbreads

Buckwheat is often mistaken for a type of wheat, but in fact it is a totally gluten-free seed. It is thought to have many healing properties, and it tastes beautiful in this recipe for flatbreads. You can find buckwheat, coconut flour and gram flour in your local health food shop.

This recipe has it all: protein, fibre and taste! It is a good one to make on a Sunday morning so that you have a batch of flatbreads ready for the week ahead – unless the rest of the family steal them from you first! **Serves 8**

2 carrots, grated
130g buckwheat flakes
400ml low fat natural yoghurt
15g Parmesan, finely grated
2 tbsp coconut flour
2 tbsp gram flour
1 tbsp goats' cheese
1 tsp baking powder
1 tsp bicarbonate of soda
1 tsp salt
Herbamare herbal salt, to taste

Preheat the oven to 180°C/350°F/gas 4 and line two baking trays with parchment paper.

Place all of the ingredients in a large bowl and use an electric mixer to beat until combined. Use a large spoon to divide the mixture evenly between the two baking trays: you should be able to fit four flatbreads on each tray. Bake for 20 minutes, then remove to cool on a wire rack. Sprinkle with Herbamare before serving.

APPROXIMATELY 100 KCAL, 1.1G FIBRE AND 3.9G PROTEIN PER SERVING

Raspberry Smoothie

This smoothie is a delicious breakfast and it takes so little time to prepare. You can make it and put it in a bottle to drink on the go – but don't leave it too long or the banana will go off.

There are lots of nutritional benefits to this smoothie. Coconut milk has the same calcium content as dairy, but with fewer calories and sugars – it is great for energy.

Flaxseed is a good source of fibre and omega-3 fatty acids. Remember that milled flaxseed needs to be kept in the fridge and really should be used up within six weeks. If you won't get through a packet in six weeks, weigh smaller portions and freeze them for later use.

Raspberries are lovely in this smoothie, but blackberries or blueberries work also. You will see that the smoothie contains frozen banana! To freeze the banana, peel it and chop it in half. Then place it in an airtight container in the freezer, where it will keep for a few months. **Serves 1 (Makes 350ml)**

100g raspberries, frozen or fresh
½ a frozen banana
250ml dairy-free coconut milk, such as Koko
1 tbsp milled flaxseed

Place the raspberries in a blender with the banana, coconut milk and flaxseed and blend until smooth and creamy.

Pour into a tall glass and serve.

APPROXIMATELY 195 KCAL, 8.2G FIBRE AND 1.9G PROTEIN PER SERVING

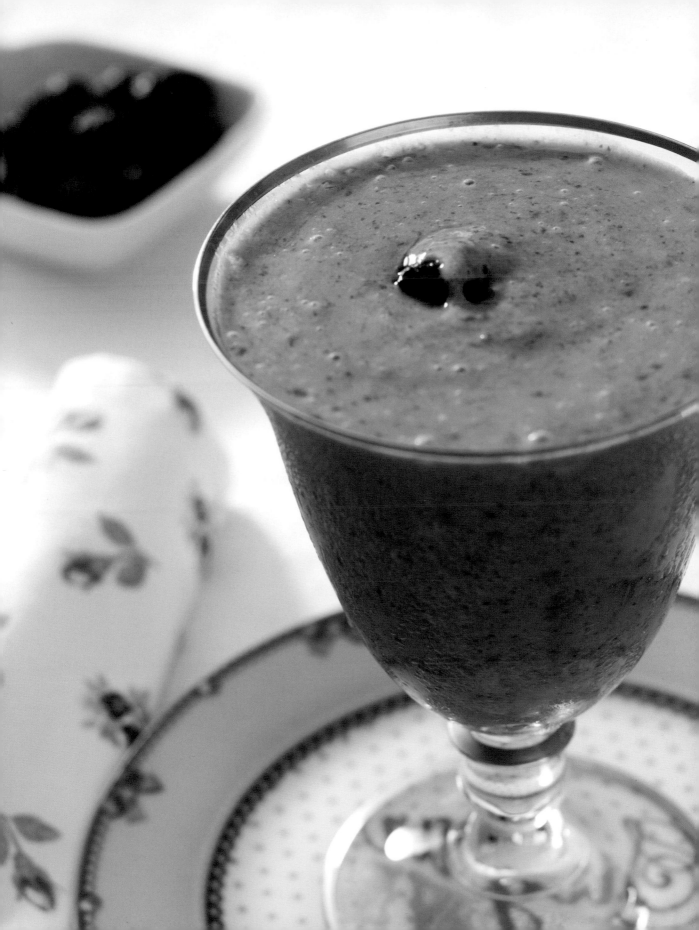

Scrambled Eggs with Caviar

This is what I call breakfast with style! Enjoy the indulgence, but don't be tempted to have any bread with this until you are closer to your goal weight. Chives give this breakfast colour and freshness, so make sure you include them. **Serves 1**

2 eggs
1 tsp butter
Salt and pepper
20g caviar
1 tsp finely chopped fresh chives

Use a whisk to lightly beat the eggs with a dash of water in a medium bowl.

Melt the butter in a non-stick frying pan and pour in the egg mixture. Cook on a low heat for 3–4 minutes, stirring frequently, until the eggs are scrambled but still nice and moist. Season and remove from the heat.

Spoon the eggs onto a warmed serving plate, top with the caviar and garnish with the chives.

APPROXIMATELY 168 KCAL AND 14.9G PROTEIN PER SERVING

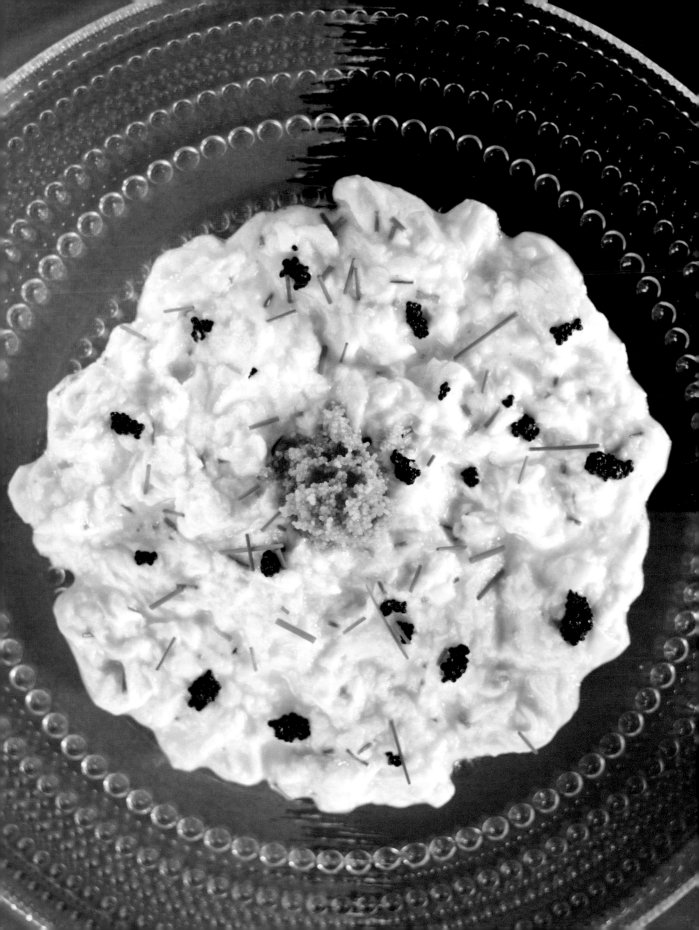

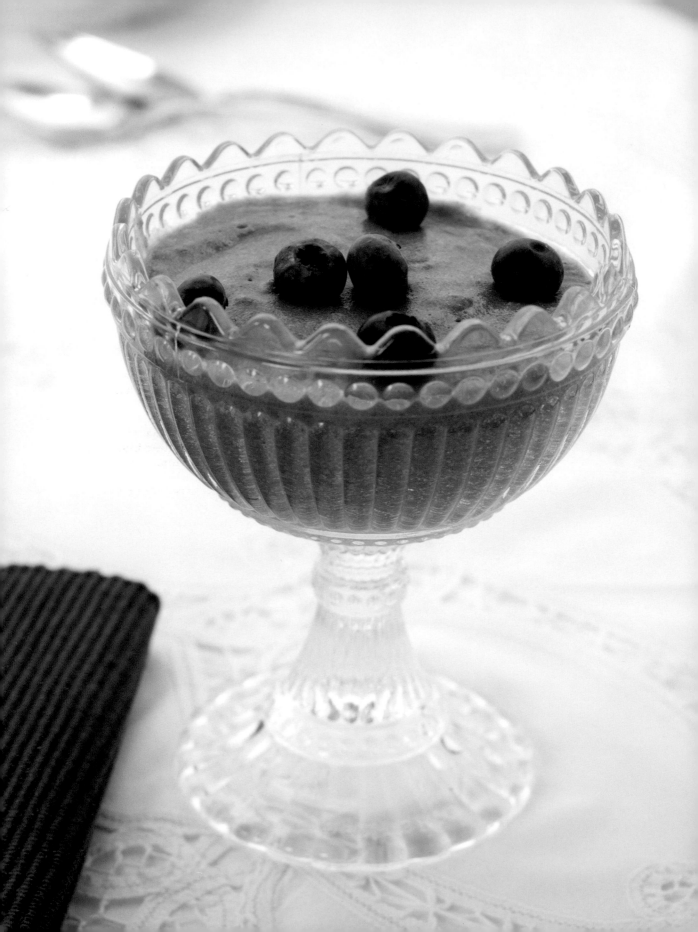

Finnish Whipped Porridge (Vispipuuro)

This is a treat! Traditionally, whipped porridge is made with a lot more sugar. Here, I've lowered the sugar so that it tastes less like a dessert and more like a delicious breakfast. You can use any berries you like. **Serves 4**

800ml water
400g berries
10g stevia
80g semolina
50ml low fat milk, to serve

Bring the water to a boil in a medium saucepan. Add the berries and stevia and simmer for 15 minutes.

Strain this mixture through a sieve into a medium bowl, pushing the berries to release their juices.

Return the hot berry juice to the saucepan, add the semolina and stir well. Cook over a low heat for 10 minutes, stirring occasionally, until the mixture has a porridge-like consistency. Remove the pan from the heat and allow it to cool (as desired).

Use an electric beater to whisk the porridge so that it becomes light and mousse-like. Spoon the mixture into serving bowls and pour a little cold milk on top.

APPROXIMATELY 147 KCAL, 2.3G FIBRE AND 4.0G PROTEIN PER SERVING

Purple 'Pick Me Up' Juice

Most people have tried juicing for health reasons, but don't forget that when juicing your fruit and vegetables you are *not* getting all the plant fibre that is so important for your health.

I have given you here a cocktail that contains a strong concentration of beta-carotene, but it is still nice enough for you to be able to drink it!

This juice might be a good breakfast for kick-starting your diet, as it will make you feel wide awake. Just make sure you plan a mid-morning snack in case the hunger pangs hit you.

You will need a juicer to make this breakfast, and all ingredients must be organic.
Serves 4 (Makes 1 litre)

4 beetroot, trimmed, scrubbed and chopped
4 carrots, trimmed, scrubbed and chopped
2 apples, washed
20g fresh ginger, peeled and chopped
½ cucumber, washed
2 celery sticks, trimmed and washed

Pass the beetroot through a juicer. Add the carrots, apples, ginger, cucumber and celery in that order.

Stir well, pour into tall glasses and serve at once.

APPROXIMATELY 143 KCAL AND 3.6G PROTEIN PER SERVING

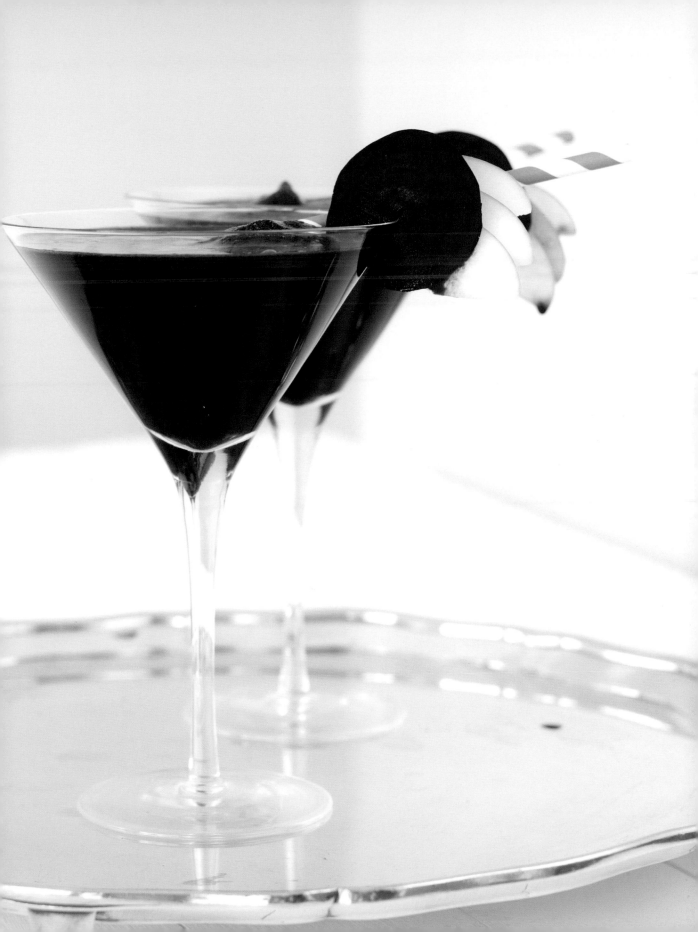

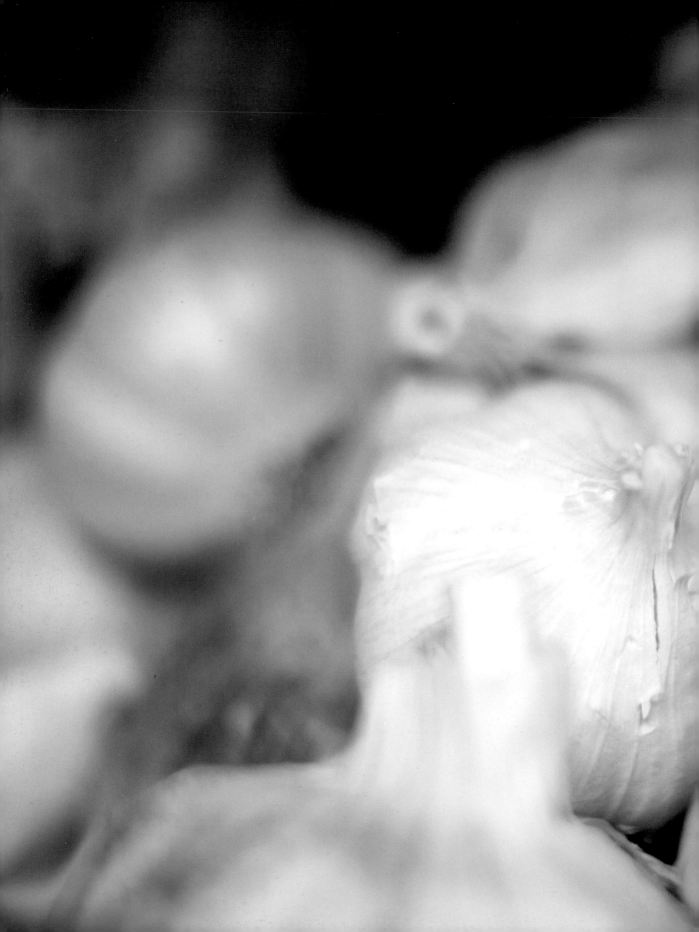

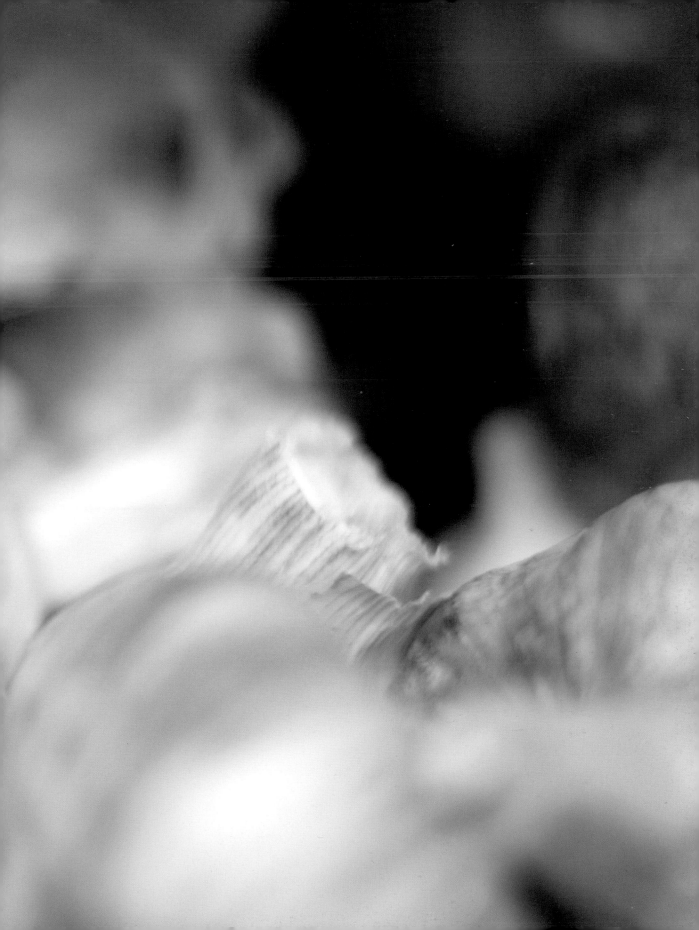

Lunch

This is probably the most challenging time of the day, as you can't just grab a sandwich without thinking about the calories. You need to be organised: failing to prepare is preparing to fail!

Get into the habit of preparing your own lunch. This will do wonders for your health and for your finances! Buying lunch out every day leaves you vulnerable to picking up other things while standing in the queue – crisps, a chocolate bar or even a bottle of wine for the evening. It's best to avoid this kind of temptation.

If you make these healthy lunches for yourself, you will soon notice the absence of the infamous afternoon slump. You just won't have that desperate craving for coffee and biscuits anymore. This in itself will help you to stay on track for the rest of the day.

If you are making lunch at home to bring to the office, invest in the best containers and flasks. This makes things convenient and hassle-free.

Remember to eat plenty of vegetables, because little side salads are not enough. Always incorporate protein: it keeps you fuller for longer. Vary your carbohydrates – try crackers, pittas, breads or wraps. With a bit of planning, lunch can always be interesting.

I insist that my patients make lots of soups. The week that a patient falls off the wagon is the week that they have no soups prepared! That is why I have included so many soups in this book. Some soups are a meal in themselves: you won't need anything else with them. Some soups are Filler Soups: they are lighter and are great for 'bulking up' your lunchtime meal. So get cooking and make use of your freezer. If you have plenty of soup stashed away, you will never face a boring lunch ever again!

Dill-Cured Salmon Tartare

Dill-cured salmon is a flavour I cherish from my childhood home. It might seem like a lot of effort, but you will love the taste! It is commonly eaten in Finland and Sweden and is typically served as an open sandwich on buttered rye bread. According to the classic recipe, you should also serve it with a raw egg yolk.

My mother often makes tartare salad with the salmon she has prepared *tuoresuolattu* (dill-cured). You don't have to dill-cure the salmon for this tartare: you can just use uncured raw salmon. If you decide to dill-cure the salmon, you must prepare it at least 24 hours ahead. In my opinion, it is worth it! **Serves 4**

FOR THE DILL-CURED SALMON
1 tsp coarse sea salt
1 tsp freshly ground black pepper
½ tsp sugar
1–2 tbsp finely chopped fresh dill
600g salmon fillet, skin on, pin bones
  removed

FOR THE TARTARE
6 shallots, finely chopped
1 scallion, finely chopped
½ small red onion, finely chopped
¼ leek, trimmed and finely chopped
1–2 tbsp finely chopped fresh dill
1–2 tbsp finely chopped fresh parsley
200g low fat crème fraîche
Finely grated rind of 1 lemon
Juice of 1 lemon
100g capers, drained and chopped
  (optional)
Salt
Freshly ground black pepper
8 round crispbreads, such as Finn Crisp
  (2 per person), to serve

For the dill-cured salmon, combine the salt, pepper, sugar and dill in a small bowl. Lay a large sheet of parchment paper on your work surface. Empty the dill mix onto the middle of the parchment paper and place the salmon on top, skin side up so that the flesh makes contact with the dill mix. Wrap the salmon, folding the parchment paper like an envelope. Place the salmon parcel on a plate and refrigerate for 12 hours. Then turn over the parcel and leave the salmon to cure for another 12 hours in the fridge.

For the tartare, remove the skin and excess salt from the dill-cured salmon. (If you are using uncured raw salmon, remove the skin and sprinkle the fillet with ½ teaspoon salt.) Finely chop the salmon fillet and place it in a medium bowl. Gently mix in the remaining tartare ingredients and season to taste. Arrange the tartare on crispbreads and serve.

APPROXIMATELY 381 KCAL, 5.2G FIBRE AND 27.6G PROTEIN PER SERVING

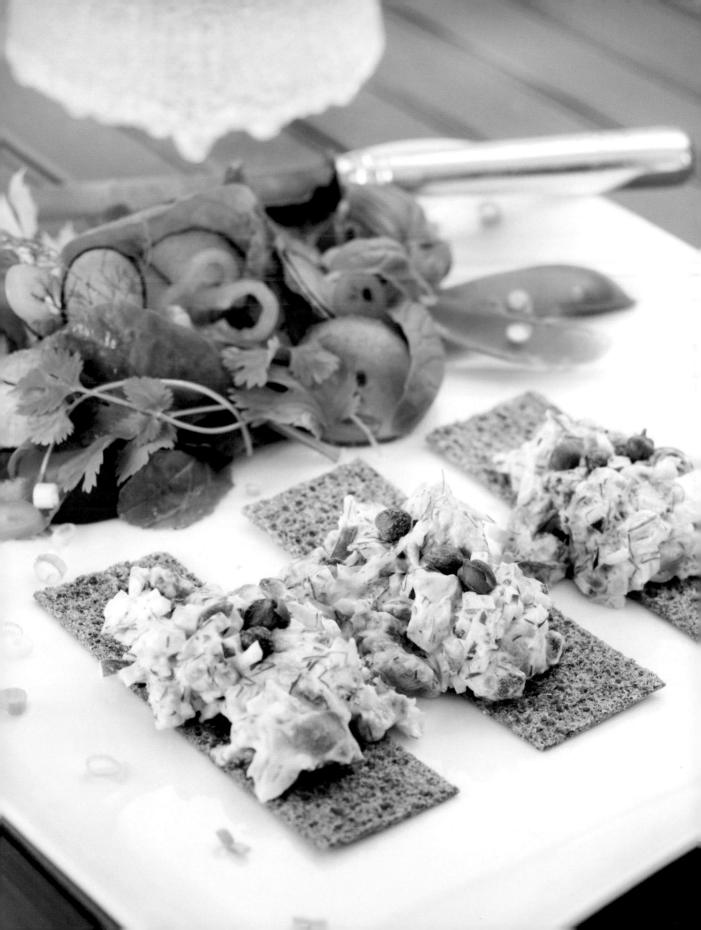

Seafood Rice Paper Rolls

Wash your hands, roll up your sleeves and try something totally different! This is a great dish to make with friends: the sauces are delicious and you'll have fun making the rolls.

This recipe uses smoked salmon but the rolls are also delicious with cooked prawns. If you really want to add flavour to this lunch, make both of the dipping sauces. **Serves 4**

FOR THE CHILLI SAUCE
½–1 red chilli, deseeded and sliced into thin strips
Juice of ½–1 lemon
1 tsp balsamic vinegar
1–2 tbsp soy sauce
½–1 tsp stevia

FOR THE PEANUT SAUCE
1 tbsp peanut butter
2 tbsp boiling water
1 tbsp soy sauce
½ tsp stevia

FOR THE SEAFOOD RICE PAPER ROLLS
160g Konnyaku glass noodles
1 carrot, peeled and finely sliced
½ cucumber, finely sliced
4 iceberg lettuce leaves, finely sliced
1 tbsp finely chopped fresh coriander
100g smoked salmon, finely sliced
8 x 20cm round rice papers

Mix all of the ingredients for the chilli sauce in a small bowl and set aside.

Mix all of the ingredients for the peanut sauce in a small bowl and set aside.

For the rice paper rolls, cook the noodles according to the packet instructions, drain and set aside. Place all of the ingredients except the rice papers into separate bowls.

Place one of the rice paper sheets into a bowl of warm water to just cover and leave for about 30 seconds, or until softened. Drain on kitchen paper. Lay some of each of the noodles, carrot, cucumber, lettuce, coriander and smoked salmon in the bottom third of the circle. Roll up and fold in the sides to create a neat parcel. The rice paper will be slightly sticky, so it will hold together.

Repeat this process with the remaining rice paper sheets and filling ingredients. Serve the rolls with the chilli and peanut dipping sauces on the side.

APPROXIMATELY 110 KCAL, 0.6G FIBRE AND 0.9G PROTEIN PER SERVING (WITH 1 TBSP SAUCE)

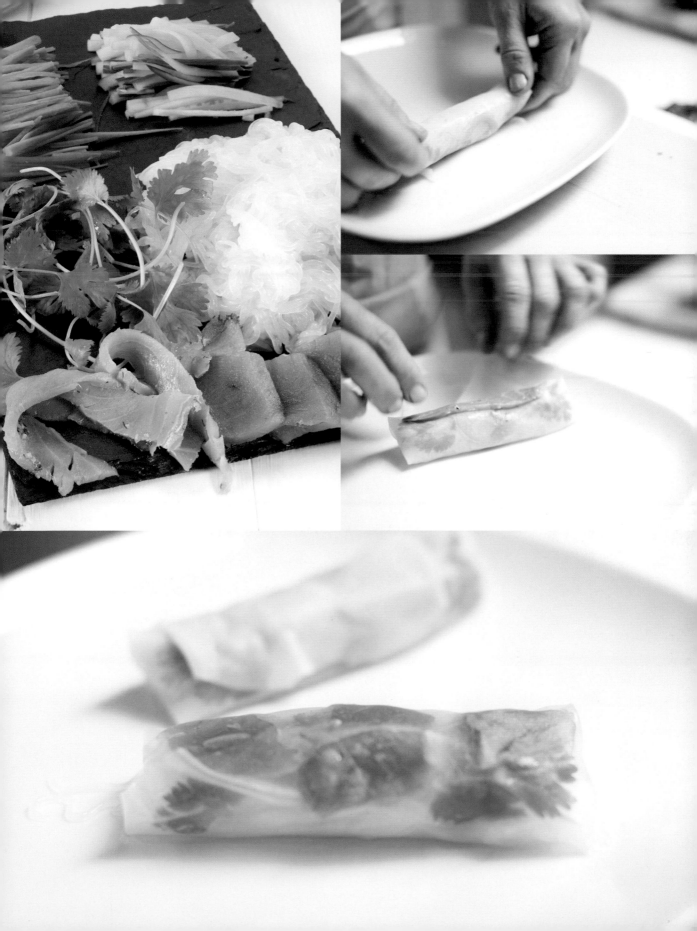

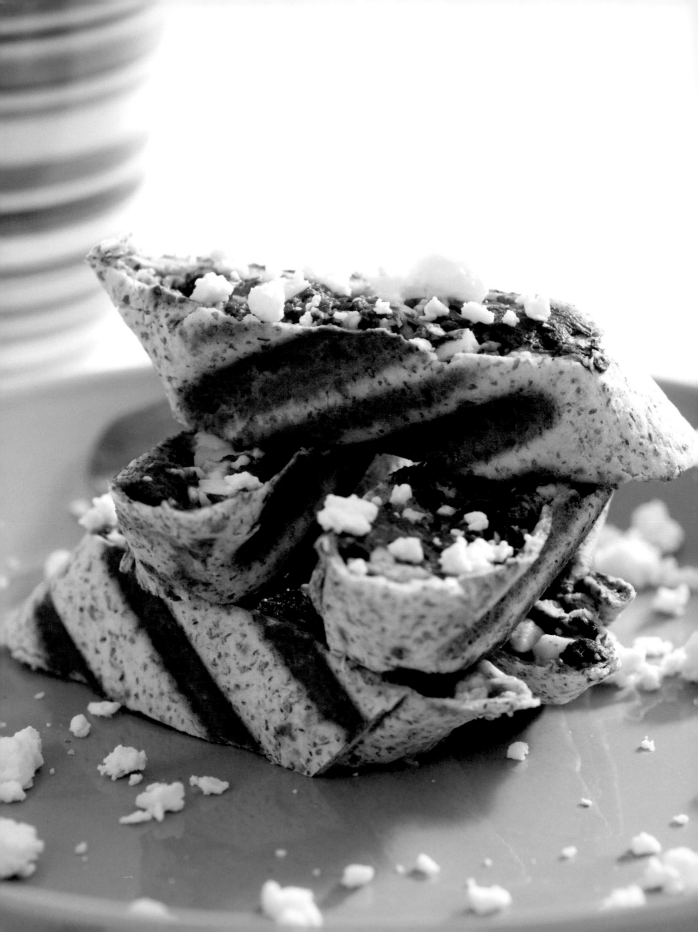

Spinach and Feta Quesadilla

This quesadilla is a lovely side dish for a Filler Soup – and spinach and feta is a classic combination. It can be hard to find wholemeal tortillas, so buy them in bulk and freeze for convenience. This recipe is really simple when you use a sandwich maker. **Serves 4**

Cooking spray
200g spinach leaves, trimmed and
  washed
200g low fat feta, cubed
2 hard-boiled eggs, peeled and chopped
Freshly ground black pepper
2 wholemeal tortillas

Lightly spray the sandwich maker wells with cooking spray and preheat.

Cook the spinach in a steamer for 3 minutes. Squeeze out the excess water and finely chop the spinach. Mix the chopped spinach, feta and eggs in a medium bowl and season with black pepper.

Divide the spinach mixture between the two tortillas. Neatly roll the individual tortillas and cook them together in the sandwich maker for about 3 minutes. Halve the cooked tortillas and serve without delay.

APPROXIMATELY 94 KCAL, 1.9G FIBRE AND 5.5G PROTEIN PER SERVING

Summer Soup

This soup is a family favourite in Finland. Traditionally it would include fresh vegetables, but if time is an issue for you, use frozen vegetables instead. That way, you have no excuses about not getting to the shop to get your soup ingredients – the only fresh vegetable you need is an onion! **Serves 8**

1 litre light soya milk
8 carrots, peeled and sliced into thin
   rounds
1 onion, finely chopped
500g cauliflower florets
400g broccoli florets
A handful of mangetout
8 radishes, thinly sliced (optional)
Freshly ground white pepper
Parmesan, to serve

Bring the milk to a boil in a large pan over a medium heat. Add the carrots and onion and cook for 5 minutes. Add the cauliflower and broccoli and cook for a further 5 minutes. Add the mangetout and radishes and cook for a further 5 minutes. The soup is ready when all of the vegetables are al dente.

Season with white pepper. Ladle the soup into warmed serving bowls, sprinkle a teaspoon of grated Parmesan over each one and serve.

APPROXIMATELY 113 KCAL, 6.9G FIBRE AND 6.8G PROTEIN PER SERVING

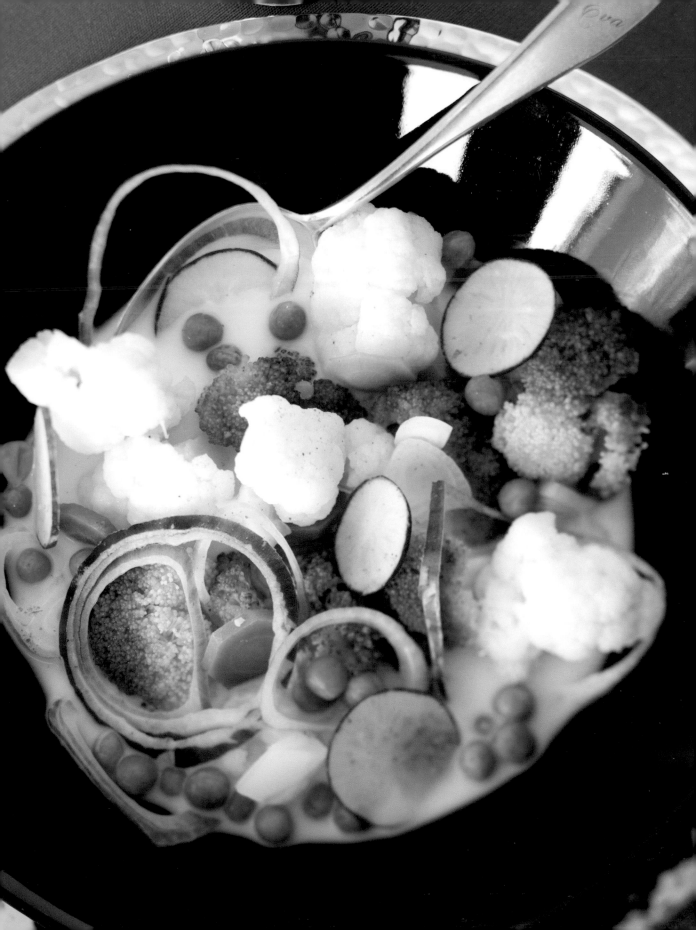

Mima's Cabbage Soup

This is my mother's recipe. Maybe she is the one to blame for my addiction to cabbage, but you can't say that's a bad thing! Make a big batch of this for the freezer and you are never stuck. **Serves 8**

1 large leek, finely sliced
1kg cabbage (green or white), shredded
1.9 litres beef or vegetable stock
½ tsp dried sage
½ tsp dried thyme
½ tsp tarragon (dried or fresh)

Heat a few tablespoons of water in a large pot over a medium heat. Add the leek and cabbage and simmer for a few minutes, until softened. Add the stock, cover and simmer for 20 minutes. Stir in the herbs and simmer, uncovered, for 3–5 minutes. Purée with a hand blender until smooth. Ladle into warmed serving bowls.

APPROXIMATELY 56 KCAL, 3.2G FIBRE AND 2.3G PROTEIN PER SERVING

Tom Yum Soup

FILLER SOUP

Don't be put off by the long list of herbs and spices: they should all be part of your store cupboard essentials. Sometimes I think that Thai ingredients are magical, since so many Thai people are so healthy and slim! **Serves 8**

1 litre vegetable stock
2 courgettes, chopped
½ cauliflower, broken into florets, stems finely chopped
3–4 slices dried galangal
4–6 kaffir lime leaves
1 stick lemongrass, outer layer discarded, inner flesh chopped roughly
1 red chilli, deseeded and finely chopped
2 tbsp soy sauce
160ml full fat coconut milk

Bring the vegetable stock to a boil in a large pan. Add the courgettes, cauliflower florets and stems, galangal, lime leaves, lemongrass and chilli. Reduce the heat and simmer until all the vegetables are soft.

Remove the galangal, lemongrass and lime leaves from the soup, then purée the soup with a hand blender until smooth. Stir in the soy sauce and coconut milk and reheat gently. Ladle into warmed serving bowls.

APPROXIMATELY 114 KCAL, 1.9G FIBRE AND 3.4G PROTEIN PER SERVING

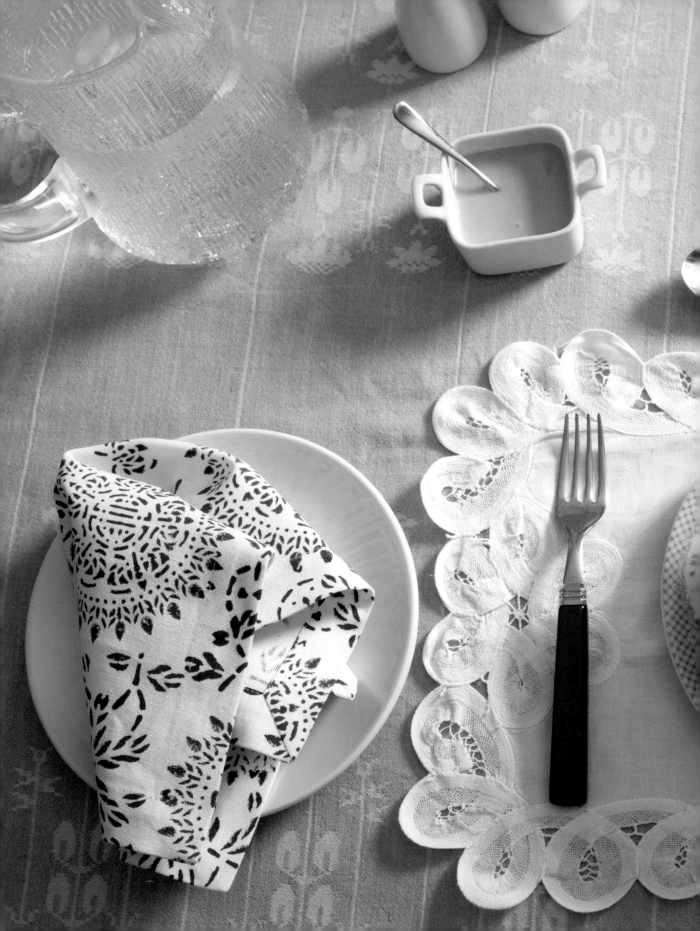

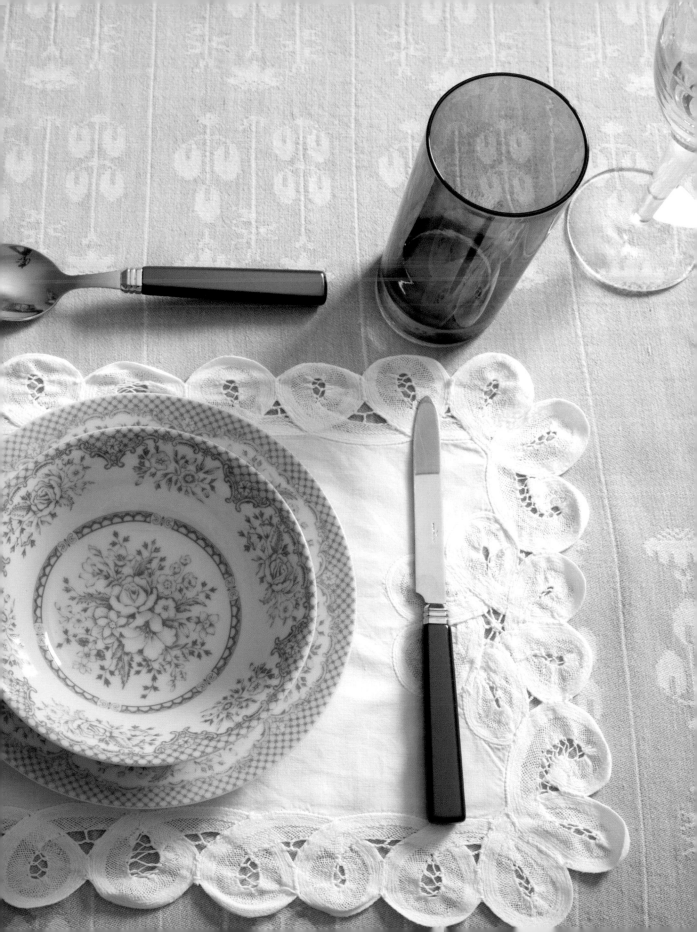

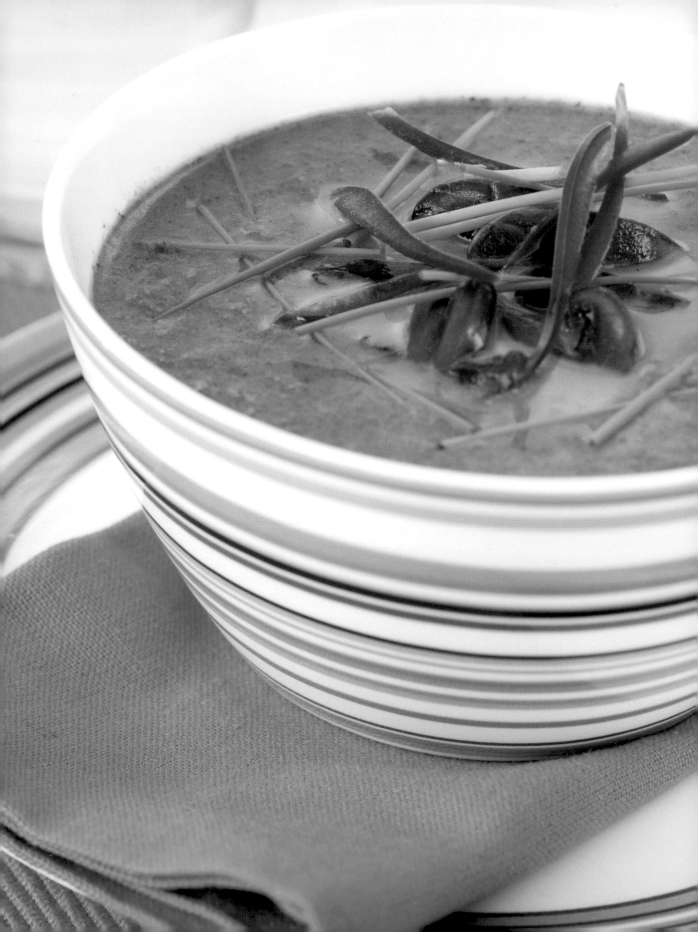

Celeriac Mushroom Soup

Celeriac is a wonderful and very versatile vegetable. Don't be put off by its somewhat ugly appearance. Actually, I once caught my puppy, Sisu, trying to eat a celeriac – I think he thought it was a football! I am not suggesting you play football with your celeriac, but you should try cooking it in any recipe that calls for turnips. **Serves 8**

1 tbsp olive oil
400g mushrooms, sliced
1 celeriac, peeled and diced
1 cauliflower, cut into small florets
2 litres mushroom stock
Salt and pepper

Heat the olive oil in a large pan over a medium heat. Fry the mushrooms for 3 minutes. Add the celeriac, cauliflower and stock and bring to the boil. Reduce the heat and simmer for 20 minutes, until the celeriac is soft.

Purée the soup with a hand blender until smooth. Season to taste, then ladle the soup into warmed serving bowls.

APPROXIMATELY 81 KCAL, 5.9G FIBRE AND 5.7G PROTEIN PER SERVING

Tomato Soup

FILLER SOUP

I use cabbage a lot in my recipes – even in this one for Tomato Soup. If you want to vary it, you could try courgette instead of cabbage and use just one specific herb, such as basil. It is delicious either way! **Serves 8**

1 tsp olive oil
4 leeks, finely sliced
200g cabbage, shredded
2 x 400g tins of whole peeled tomatoes
2 garlic cloves, crushed
1 tbsp finely chopped fresh herbs
1.5 litres vegetable stock
1 tsp sugar or stevia
Freshly ground black pepper
Crème fraîche, to serve (optional)

Heat the olive oil in a large pan over a medium heat. Add the leeks and fry gently for 3–5 minutes. Add the cabbage, tomatoes, garlic, herbs and stock and bring to the boil. Reduce the heat and simmer for 20 minutes.

When the vegetables have cooked through, purée with a hand blender until smooth. Stir in the sugar and season with black pepper. Ladle the soup into warmed serving bowls and top each one with a teaspoon of crème fraîche.

APPROXIMATELY 97 KCAL, 6.4G FIBRE AND 5.1G PROTEIN PER SERVING

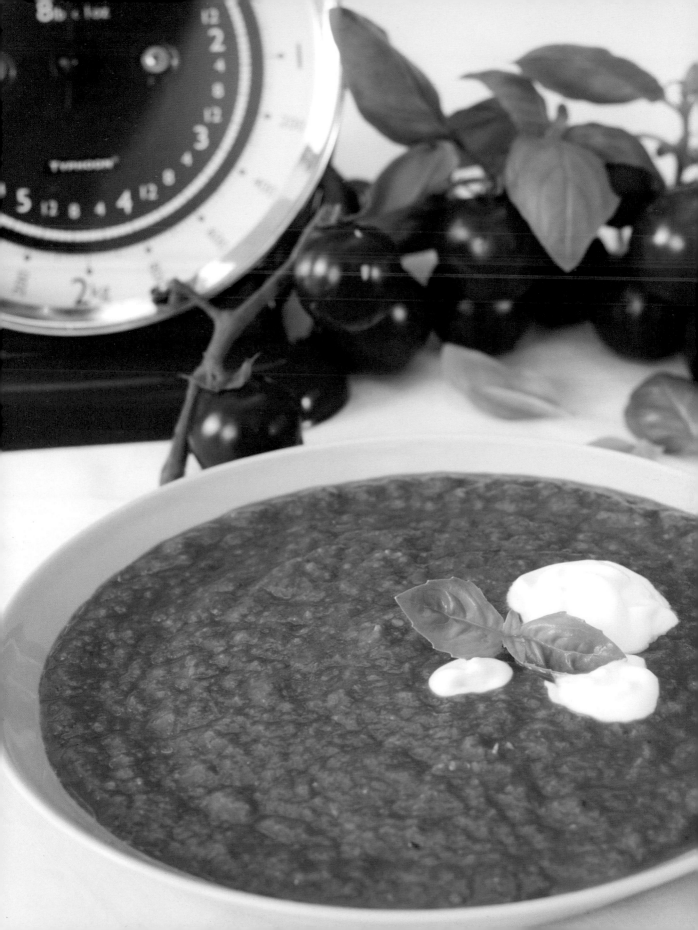

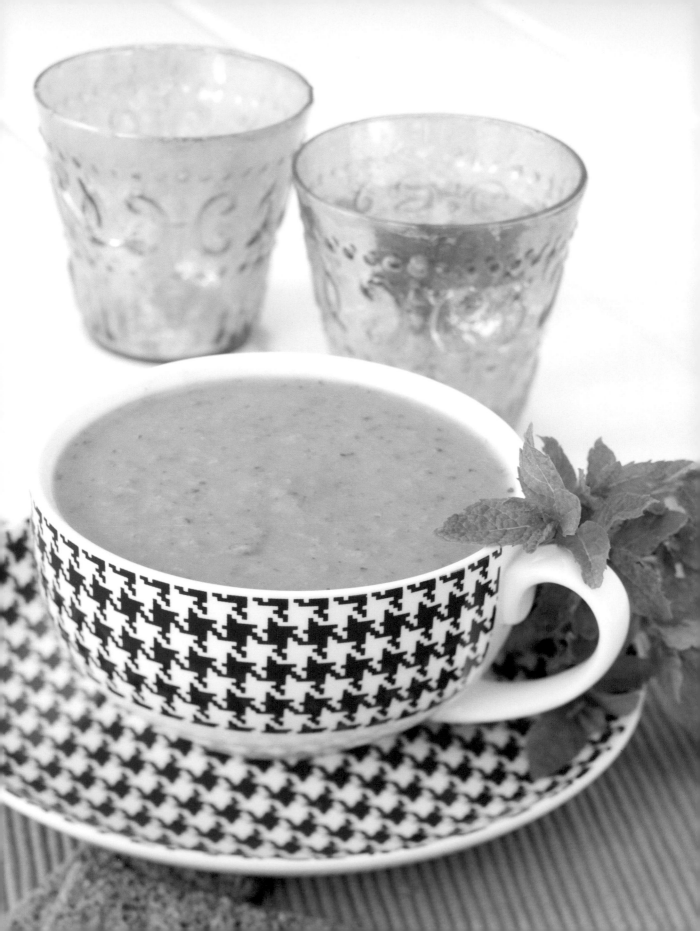

Pea and Mint Soup

FILLER SOUP

Peas have such a lovely colour and a lot of fibre. Children are also big fans of this soup. You could try this recipe without the mint, adding some wasabi instead. **Serves 8**

2 tsp olive oil
½ leek, finely sliced
1kg courgettes, finely chopped
200g frozen peas
1.3 litres vegetable stock
4 tbsp finely chopped fresh mint
Freshly ground white pepper

Heat the olive oil in a large pan over a low heat. Add the leeks and cook for 3 minutes. Add the courgettes and cook for a further 3 minutes. Add the peas and stock and bring to the boil. Reduce the heat and simmer for 15 minutes, until the courgettes are soft.

Remove from the heat and add the mint leaves, then purée with a hand blender until smooth. Season with white pepper and ladle the soup into warmed serving bowls.

APPROXIMATELY 98 KCAL, 4.7G FIBRE AND 5.6G PROTEIN PER SERVING

Celery Roquefort Soup

FILLER SOUP

If you have the time and patience, sauté the vegetables first to soften them a little. This is a soup I make when I have a craving for the lovely creamy soups in restaurants! **Serves 8**

1 tbsp olive oil
500g celery, finely sliced
1 large leek, finely sliced
1 litre vegetable stock
1 tbsp soy sauce
50g Roquefort, crumbled
Freshly ground black pepper

Heat the olive oil in a large pan over a medium heat. Add the celery and leek and fry for 3–5 minutes. Add the stock, soy sauce and Roquefort. Stir well, reduce the heat and simmer for 20 minutes.

Season with black pepper. If you prefer a creamy consistency, purée the soup with a hand blender until smooth. If not, simply ladle the soup into warmed serving bowls.

APPROXIMATELY 101 KCAL, 3.0G FIBRE AND 4.0G PROTEIN PER SERVING

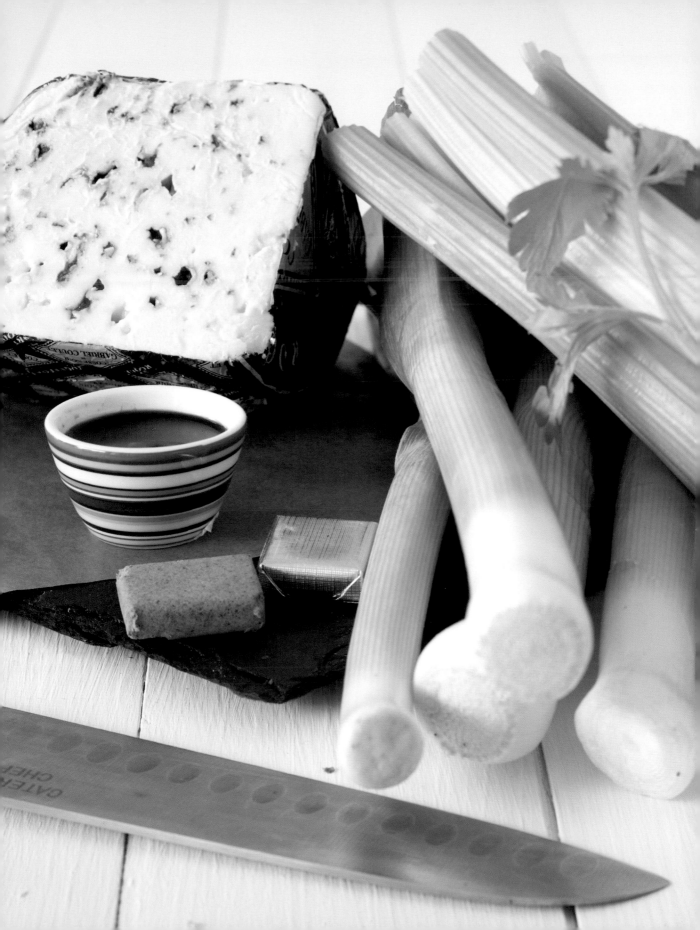

Thai Mushroom Soup

FILLER SOUP

I have recently started using coconut oil in a lot of my recipes because of its lovely sweet flavour. It also has a very high smoking point and is therefore good for stir-fries and other high-heat cooking methods. As it is solid at room temperature, buy it in jars rather than bottles. **Serves 8**

1 tbsp coconut oil
1 tbsp yellow curry paste (or less, if it's too spicy for you)
1 shallot, finely chopped
1 large courgette, finely chopped
750g chestnut mushrooms, sliced
2 litres mushroom stock
2 tsp fish sauce
1 tsp sugar or stevia
160ml coconut milk
Freshly ground white pepper

Heat the coconut oil in a large pan over a low heat. Add the curry paste and shallot and fry gently for 2 minutes. Add the courgette and mushrooms, cover with the stock and bring to the boil. Cook for 15 minutes.

Remove a few spoons of mushrooms from the soup and set aside. Purée the soup with a hand blender until smooth. Stir in the fish sauce, sugar and coconut milk. Return the cooked mushrooms to the pan and reheat gently. Season with white pepper and ladle into warmed serving bowls.

APPROXIMATELY 174 KCAL, 2.9G FIBRE AND 9.0G PROTEIN PER SERVING

Tricolour Soup

 FILLER SOUP

Everybody loves a carrot soup. I've added other vegetables here to reduce the overall carbohydrate content – and to make an Irish tricolour! This soup freezes very well, so get those containers out and free yourself from the kitchen for one day. **Serves 8**

½ tbsp olive oil
2 turkey rashers, sliced
½ onion, finely sliced
3 large carrots, peeled and chopped
1 courgette, chopped
½ cauliflower, broken into small florets
500ml vegetable or beef stock
Freshly ground white pepper

Heat the olive oil in a large pan over a medium heat. Add the turkey rashers and fry for 3 minutes. Use a slotted spoon to remove the cooked turkey rashers from the pan and set aside.

Now add the onion to the pan and fry for 3–5 minutes. Add the carrots, courgette, cauliflower and stock and bring to the boil. Reduce the heat and simmer for 20 minutes, until all the vegetables are tender.

Return the cooked turkey rashers to the pan and purée the soup with a hand blender until smooth. Season with white pepper and ladle the soup into warmed serving bowls.

APPROXIMATELY 88 KCAL, 4.6G FIBRE AND 6.3G PROTEIN PER SERVING

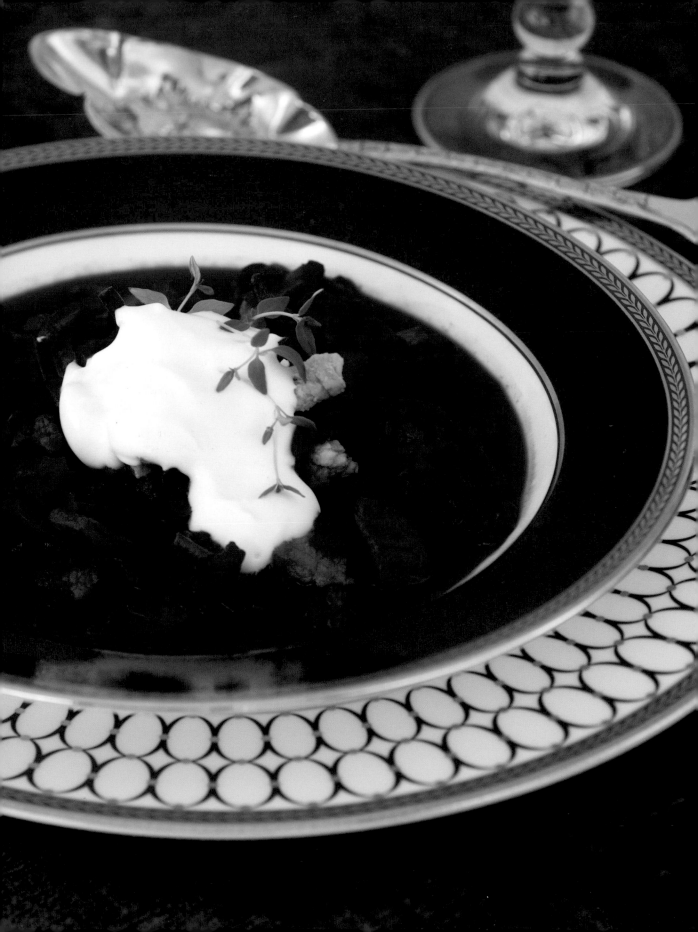

Borscht

My grandfather brought some of his Russian traditions to our family kitchen. This soup is one of them. Smetana is available in the Polish sections of Irish supermarkets, but you can use low fat soured cream instead.

And remember: don't rush to your doctor if your urine turns purple after eating this soup. This is all normal when you eat beetroot! **Serves 4**

1 tsp olive oil
300g turkey rashers, sliced
2 onions, finely sliced
3 carrots, peeled and diced
2 beetroot, peeled and diced; plus 1
   beetroot, peeled and coarsely grated
1 celery stick, diced
250g white cabbage, shredded
1.25 litres beef stock
1 tbsp red wine vinegar
Freshly ground black pepper
Smetana or soured cream

Heat the olive oil in a large pan over a medium heat. Add the turkey rashers and fry for 3–5 minutes. Use a slotted spoon to remove the cooked turkey from the pan and set aside.

Add the onions to the pan and fry for 3 minutes. Add the carrots, diced beetroot, celery and cabbage (leaving aside the grated beetroot for now). Pour in the beef stock, stir well and reduce the heat. Simmer for 30–40 minutes, until all the vegetables are tender.

Return the cooked turkey to the pan. Add the vinegar and grated beetroot. Stir well and season with black pepper. Ladle the soup into warmed serving bowls and top each one with a tablespoon of smetana.

APPROXIMATELY 357 KCAL, 8.1G FIBRE AND 32.6G PROTEIN PER SERVING

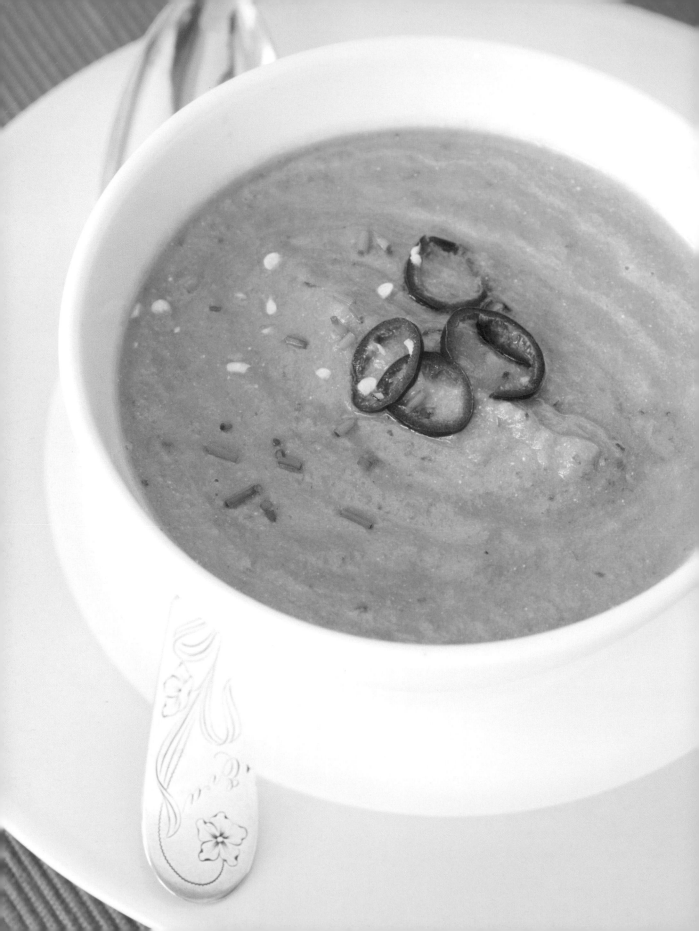

Creamy Chorizo Soup

Even a small piece of chorizo adds such an amazing flavour to this soup. It is worth taking out the visible fat pieces, though. Believe me – the flavour won't suffer!
Serves 4

2 tsp butter
50g chorizo, peeled, halved lengthways, with any visible fat scooped out (35g net weight)
½ leek, finely sliced
1–2 cloves garlic, crushed
1 small red pepper, finely chopped
1 small yellow pepper, finely chopped
4 courgettes, finely chopped
1 small carrot, peeled and finely chopped
½ red chilli, deseeded and finely chopped (optional)
1.25 litres chicken stock
60g soured cream
Freshly ground white pepper

Heat the butter in a large pan over a low heat. Gently fry the chorizo, leek and garlic for 3–5 minutes. Add a little vegetable stock if they start sticking to the pan.

Add the peppers, courgettes, carrot, chilli and chicken stock. Stir well and bring to the boil. Reduce the heat and simmer for 20 minutes.

When the vegetables have cooked through, purée with a hand blender until smooth. Stir in the soured cream and reheat gently. Season with white pepper and ladle into warmed serving bowls.

APPROXIMATELY 134 KCAL, 2.2G FIBRE AND 6.1G PROTEIN PER SERVING

Russian Soup (Solyanka)

I like to bring some of my family history and traditions into my soups. In this recipe, I have been inspired by Solyanka – a thick, tomato-based Russian stew that contains different meats and chopped pickles. My version uses smoked ham, which is full of flavour. **Serves 4**

500g piece of raw smoked ham
1 tbsp butter
1 leek, finely sliced
2 carrots, peeled and diced
1 large parsnip, peeled and diced
1 turnip, peeled and diced
200g cabbage, shredded
4 garlic cloves, finely chopped
400g tin of chopped tomatoes
70g tomato purée
2 bay leaves
1 tsp black peppercorns
1 litre vegetable stock
1 pickled gherkin, diced; plus 200ml
    liquid from the jar of pickled gherkins
    (or 200ml apple cider vinegar)
Smetana or low fat soured cream

Place the ham in a large pan of cold water, bring to the boil and skim off any impurities. Leave to simmer for 30 minutes, then drain and rinse under cold water. Allow the ham to cool and then cut it into cubes. (It will cook fully in the soup.)

Heat the butter in a very large pan over a medium heat. Add the leek and fry gently for 3 minutes. Add the carrots, parsnip, turnip, cabbage, garlic, tomatoes, tomato purée, bay leaves, peppercorns and stock. Return the cooked ham to the pot and bring to the boil. Reduce the heat, cover and simmer for 40–45 minutes, until the vegetables and ham are cooked through.

Stir in the gherkins and their juice and reheat gently. Ladle into warmed serving bowls and top each one with a tablespoon of smetana.

APPROXIMATELY 319 KCAL, 9.4G FIBRE AND 27.8G PROTEIN PER SERVING

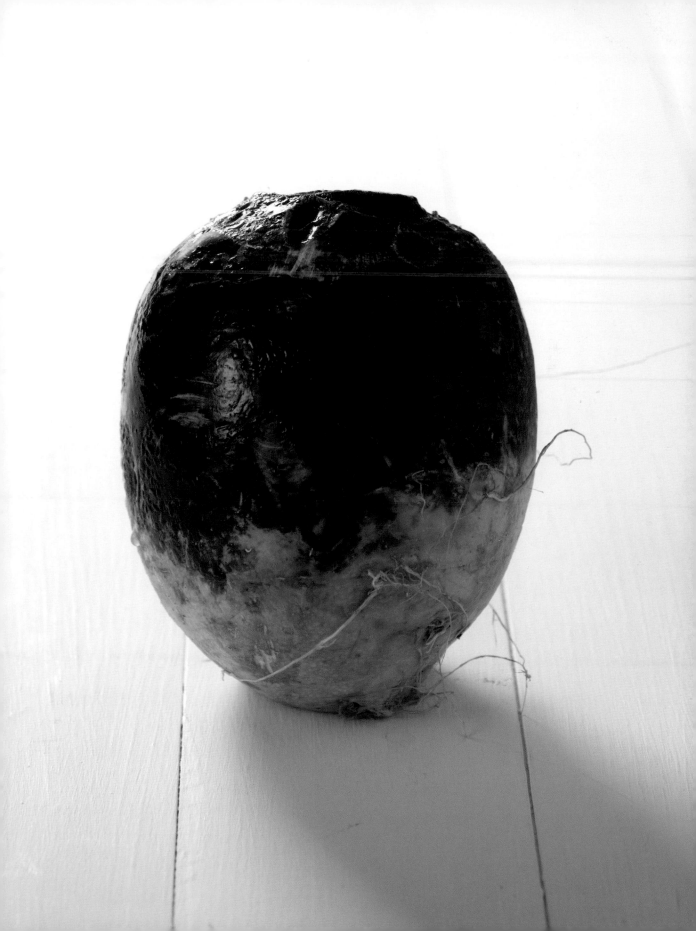

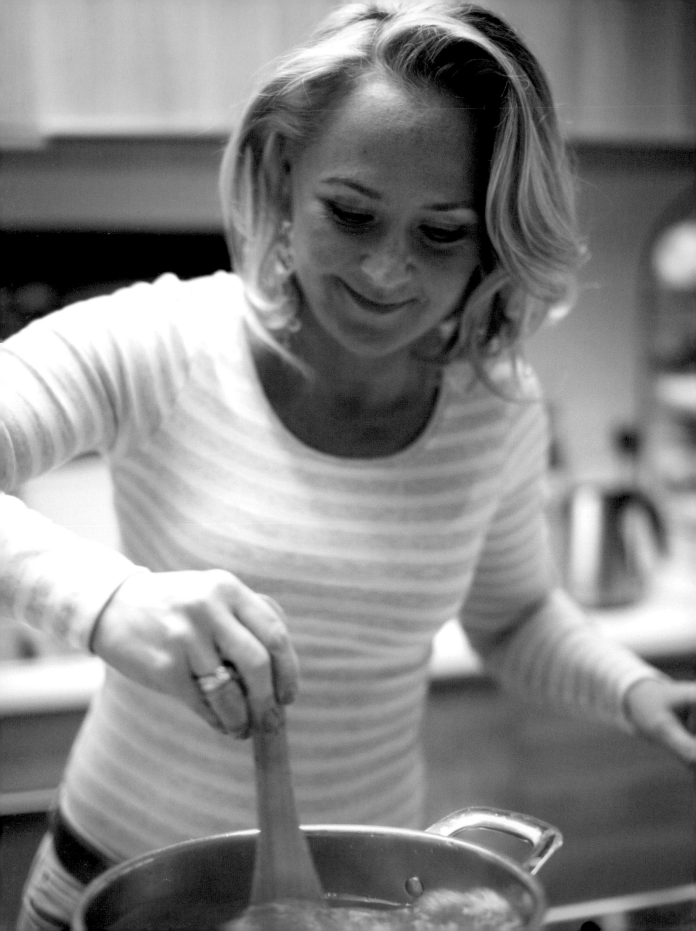

Pork Sausage Soup
(Siskonmakkarakeitto)

Traditionally this soup is one that people either love or hate, but that is because of the type of sausage we use in Finland. Here you can use either flavoured or unflavoured sausages, depending on your taste buds. Parsnips, potatoes and sausages together prepare you for a hunger-free afternoon! **Serves 4**

1 tsp olive oil
6 carrots, peeled and sliced into thin rounds
1 large onion, finely chopped
2 medium potatoes, peeled and diced
1 large parsnip, peeled and sliced into thin rounds
1.5 litres beef stock
450g flavoured pork sausages, skins removed with scissors (garlic or basil flavouring is especially nice)

Heat the olive oil in a large pan over a medium heat. Fry the carrots and onion for about 4 minutes. Add the potatoes, parsnip and stock and bring to the boil. Add the skinned sausages, cover, reduce the heat and simmer for 30–40 minutes. When the sausages and vegetables are cooked through, ladle the soup into warmed serving bowls.

APPROXIMATELY 306 KCAL, 7.6G FIBRE AND 9.6G PROTEIN PER SERVING

Fish Soup

This recipe is a really easy way to get more fish in your diet. You can find fish pie mix in most good supermarkets – it's a selection of boneless pieces of salmon and smoked/unsmoked white fish that's already prepared and ready to go into fish soups or stews.

I love the mixture of potatoes and celeriac in this recipe. By using this combination, I've been able to reduce the carbohydrate portion. You really do need fish stock for this soup, so I hope you can find it in your local shop! **Serves 4**

1 tbsp butter
1 large leek, finely sliced
½ red pepper, finely sliced
2–4 garlic cloves, crushed
400g fish pie mix
1.5 litres fish stock
½ lemon, sliced
4 small potatoes, peeled and diced
1 celeriac, peeled and diced
10g dill, leaves removed and finely chopped
2 scallions, finely sliced
1 tbsp sweet chilli sauce
2 tbsp finely chopped fresh parsley
Salt and freshly ground white pepper

Heat the butter in a large pan over a low heat. Add the leek, pepper and garlic and fry gently for 3–5 minutes. Add the fish pie mix, stock and lemon slices and stir well. Simmer for 10 minutes and skim off any impurities.

When the fish has cooked through, use a slotted spoon to remove it and set aside. Remove the lemon slices and discard them. Now add the potatoes and celeriac to the pan, cover and leave to simmer for about 25 minutes. Meanwhile, use a fork to flake the cooked fish and set aside.

When the vegetables are tender, purée the soup with a hand blender until smooth. Stir in the dill, scallions, sweet chilli sauce, parsley and flaked fish. Reheat gently and check the seasoning. Then ladle the soup into warmed serving bowls.

APPROXIMATELY 271 KCAL, 5.5G FIBRE AND 24.0G PROTEIN PER SERVING

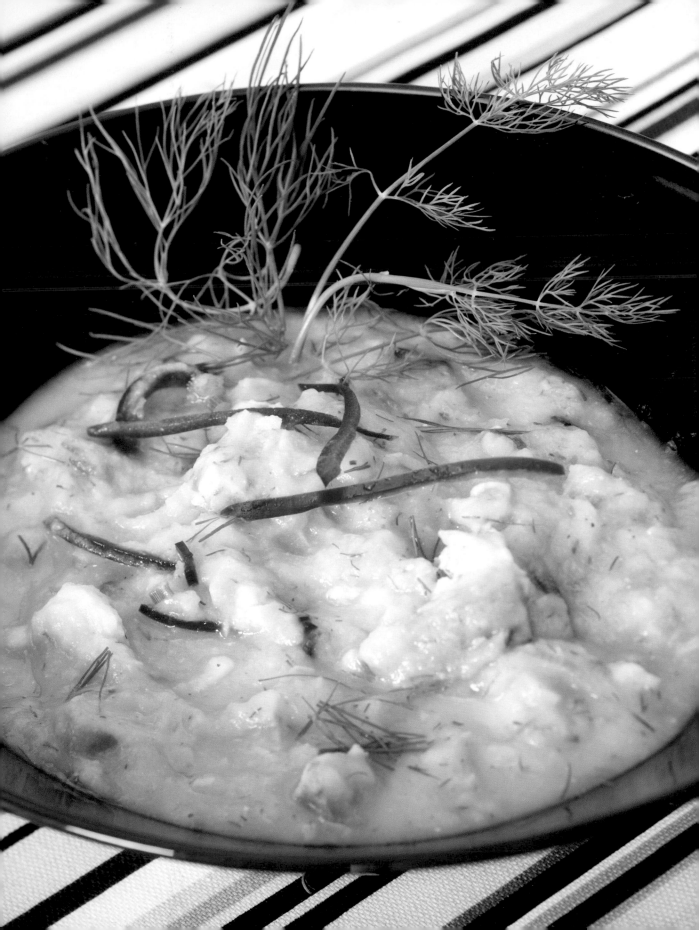

Chinese Chicken Soup

I love Asian flavours, but Asian broth-style soups feel to me like they're missing a bit of bulk. In this soup, I've used chicken and a nice mix of vegetables – and you know we all need to eat our fibre to stay full.

Don't be afraid to try some other vegetables here: green peppers instead of carrots, or some mushrooms instead of baby corn. This soup goes really well with Konnyaku noodles. **Serves 4**

FOR THE CHICKEN
4 skinless chicken breast fillets, sliced
  into thin strips
3 tbsp soy sauce
2 tbsp sesame oil
1 tbsp rice vinegar
1 tbsp maple syrup
3 tbsp Ginger Garlic Paste (p.195)
3 tbsp tahini
¼ tsp red chilli powder

FOR THE SOUP
2 tbsp sesame oil
3 large scallions, finely sliced
⅓ Irish sweetheart cabbage, shredded
1 litre chicken stock
4 carrots, peeled and sliced into thin
  rounds
190g baby corn
220g beansprouts

Place the chicken strips, soy sauce, sesame oil, rice vinegar, maple syrup, Ginger Garlic Paste, tahini and chilli powder in a medium bowl. Stir well and set aside while you cook the vegetables.

Heat the sesame oil in a large pan (or wok) over a medium heat. Add the scallions and cabbage and stir-fry for about 3 minutes. Lower the heat and add the chicken strips and their marinade. Pour in the stock, add the carrots and stir well to combine. Leave to simmer for 15 minutes.

Add the baby corn and simmer for a further 5 minutes, until tender. Stir in the beansprouts and allow them to heat through. (You can cook the beansprouts for a few more minutes if you don't want them too crunchy.) Ladle the soup into warmed serving bowls.

APPROXIMATELY 274 KCAL, 6.1G FIBRE AND 26.9G PROTEIN PER SERVING

Leek and Potato Soup

Leek and potato soup is a classic. I've added some celery to reduce the carbohydrates, but you wouldn't know this by the taste! The protein content of this soup is surprisingly high, so it should make you feel full. You can serve this soup piping hot or well chilled. **Serves 4**

1 tbsp butter
5 shallots, finely chopped
2 leeks, finely sliced
3 celery stalks, finely chopped
1 garlic clove, crushed
4 potatoes, peeled and diced
750ml chicken stock
200ml low fat crème fraîche
2 tbsp finely chopped fresh chives, to garnish
40g Parmesan, grated (optional)

Melt the butter in a large pan over a low heat. Add the shallots, leeks, celery and garlic and stir well. Cover and cook for 15 minutes, stirring occasionally, until the vegetables are softened but not browned.

Add the potatoes and stock to the pan and bring to the boil. Reduce the heat and leave to simmer, covered, for about 20 minutes.

Purée the soup with a hand blender until smooth. Stir in the crème fraîche and reheat gently. Ladle the soup into warmed serving bowls and top each one with some chives and grated Parmesan.

APPROXIMATELY 238 KCAL, 4.9G FIBRE AND 9.5G PROTEIN PER SERVING

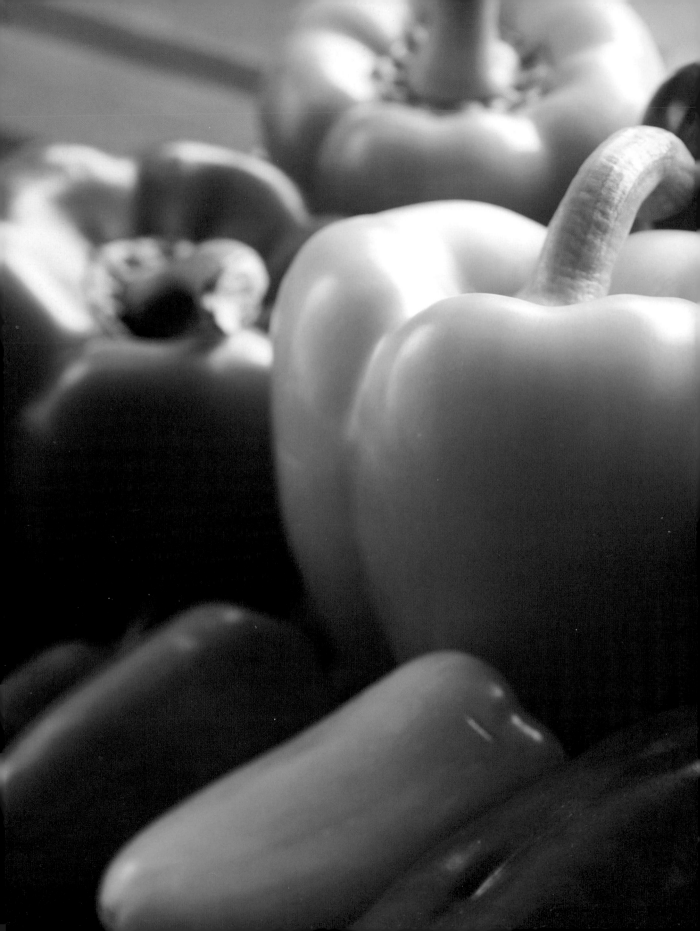

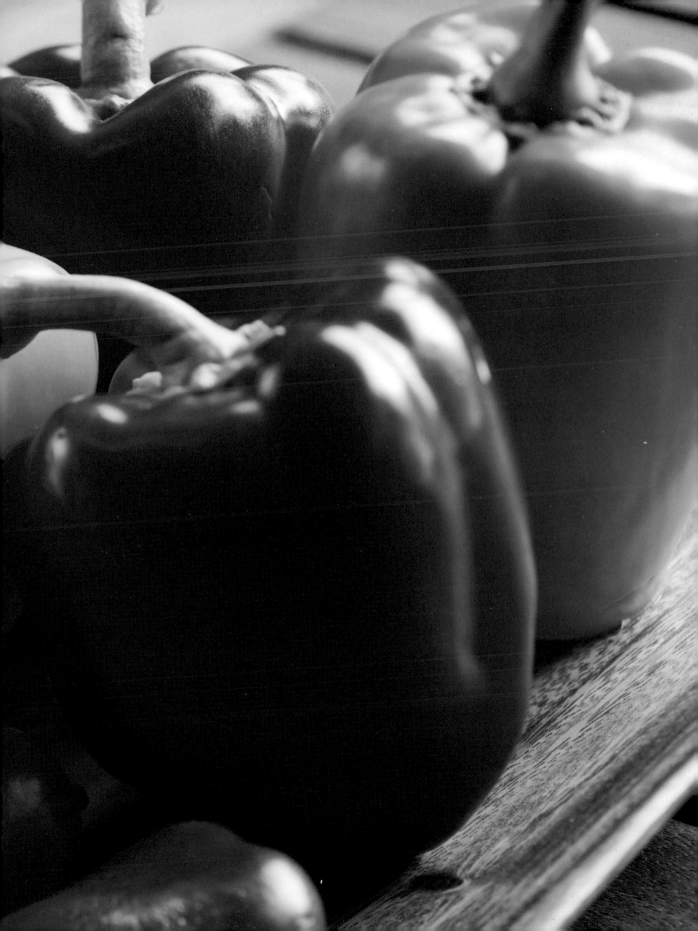

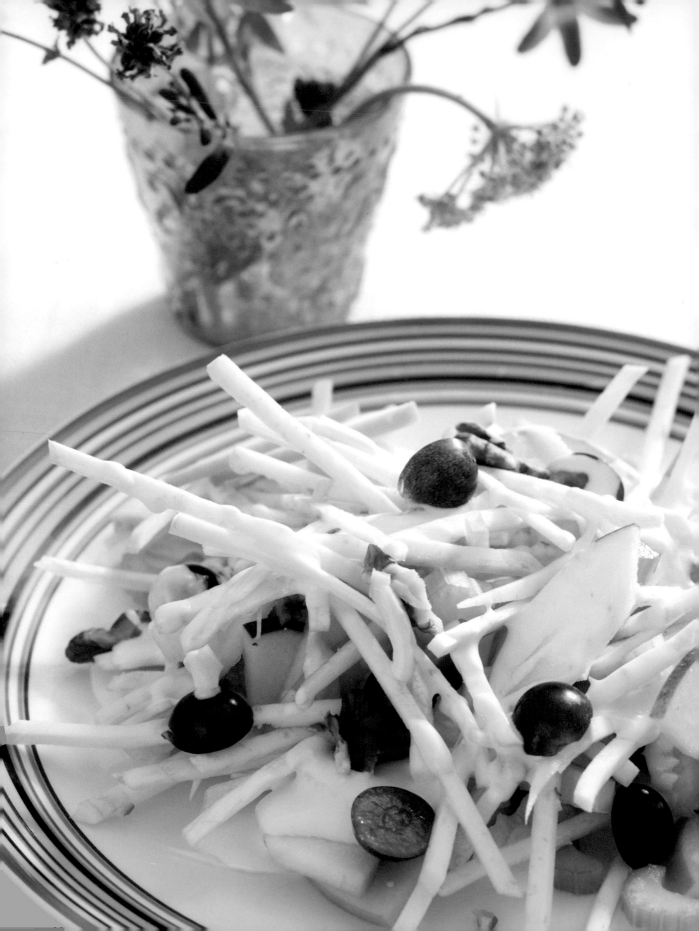

Waldorf Salad

My son couldn't believe that this salad dressing had anchovies in it! They are a very important part of the flavour – so even if you don't eat them normally, try them in this dressing. I guarantee you'll be just as surprised as he was. **Serves 4**

FOR THE DRESSING
4 tbsp low fat mayonnaise
4 tbsp low fat natural yoghurt
1 tbsp horseradish sauce
3 tbsp orange juice
4 anchovies, drained of oil and finely
   chopped

½ celeriac, peeled and cut into julienne
   strips
3 celery sticks, finely sliced
2 red apples, grated
3 tbsp raisins (or a handful of grapes,
   halved)
25g walnuts

Combine all the ingredients for the dressing in a jar with a lid and shake to combine.

Mix the celeriac, celery, apples, raisins and walnuts in a large salad bowl. Drizzle the dressing on top, mix well and serve.

APPROXIMATELY 258 KCAL, 4.4G FIBRE AND 5.5G PROTEIN PER SERVING

Warm Halloumi Salad

Preparation is the key to successful weightloss journeys. This salad can be partially prepared the evening before by roasting the butternut and beetroot while you're cooking something else in the oven. Also, one important thing I learned while living in Italy: invest in good balsamic vinegar! **Serves 4**

FOR THE DRESSING
250g blueberries
2 tbsp balsamic vinegar
2 tbsp orange juice

300g butternut squash, peeled, deseeded
    and cubed
Olive oil
Freshly ground black pepper
2 small beetroot, peeled and cubed
50g halloumi cheese, sliced
450g baby spinach
1 red onion, finely sliced
4 hard-boiled eggs, sliced

Preheat the oven to 180°C/350°F/gas 4.

Place the blueberries in a blender with the balsamic vinegar and orange juice and blend until smooth.

Brush the butternut pieces with 1 teaspoon of olive oil and some black pepper and roast for 10 minutes. Meanwhile, brush the beetroot pieces with 1 teaspoon of olive oil and some black pepper.

Add the beetroot to the butternut on the roasting tray and stir well. Roast the vegetables together for another 15 minutes.

Meanwhile, heat 1 teaspoon of olive oil in a non-stick pan over a medium heat. Fry the halloumi slices for 2 minutes on each side. Remove the halloumi from the pan and keep warm.

Arrange the spinach and red onion on a serving platter. Add the roasted butternut and beetroot and the egg slices. Top with the warm halloumi and drizzle over the dressing. Serve without delay.

APPROXIMATELY 196 KCAL, 8.5G FIBRE AND 11.3G PROTEIN PER SERVING

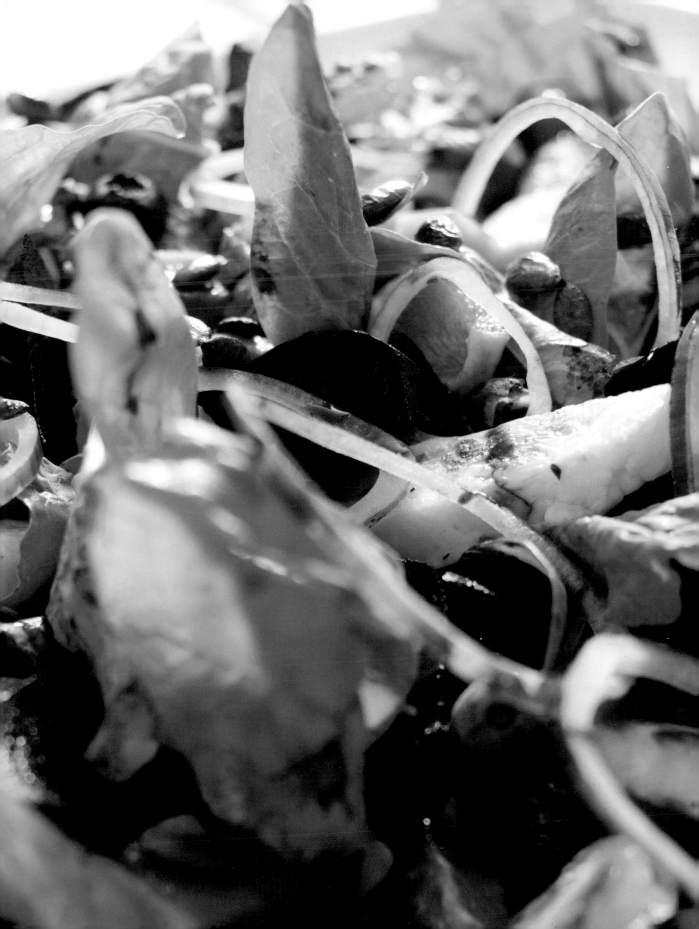

Tex-Mex Salad

This salad includes a Tex-Mex salsa, and the recipe makes more than you actually need. So use the leftover salsa to spice up any of your other dinners that need a bit of heat!

Remember to handle the jalapeño peppers carefully: use gloves and wash your hands thoroughly afterwards. **Serves 4**

FOR THE SALSA
400g tin of chopped tomatoes
100g green jalapeño peppers, roughly chopped
2 garlic cloves
½ onion, roughly chopped
½ tsp salt
½ tsp sugar
Juice of ½ lemon

FOR THE BEEF
1 tbsp olive oil
600g lean minced beef (max 10% fat)
10 cherry tomatoes, halved
Salt and freshly ground black pepper

FOR THE SALAD
1 iceberg lettuce, shredded
1 ripe avocado, peeled and diced
200g tin of sweetcorn, drained
1 small red onion, finely sliced

FOR THE QUESADILLAS
2 wholemeal tortillas
2 low fat Cheddar slices

Place all of the ingredients for the salsa in a food processor and blitz until combined. Set aside while you cook the beef.

Heat the olive oil in a large pan over a medium heat. Fry the beef until browned. Add the cherry tomatoes and a little seasoning. Stir in 2–3 tablespoons of the salsa. Cook for about 15 minutes, stirring occasionally.

Now prepare the salad. Mix the iceberg lettuce, avocado, sweetcorn and red onion in a medium bowl. Divide the salad between four serving plates.

A few minutes before serving, prepare the quesadillas. Lay one tortilla in a non-stick frying pan and top with the Cheddar slices. Place the other tortilla on top and press down gently. Place the pan on a medium heat and cook the quesadilla for 2–3 minutes on each side, until the Cheddar has melted. Cut the quesadilla into quarters and keep it warm while you prepare to serve.

Taste the beef and sauce and adjust the seasoning (you might need more black pepper). Spoon equal amounts of the beef and sauce on top of the salad on the serving plates. Top each plate with a quesadilla quarter and serve.

APPROXIMATELY 488 KCAL, 7.5G FIBRE AND 39.4G PROTEIN PER SERVING

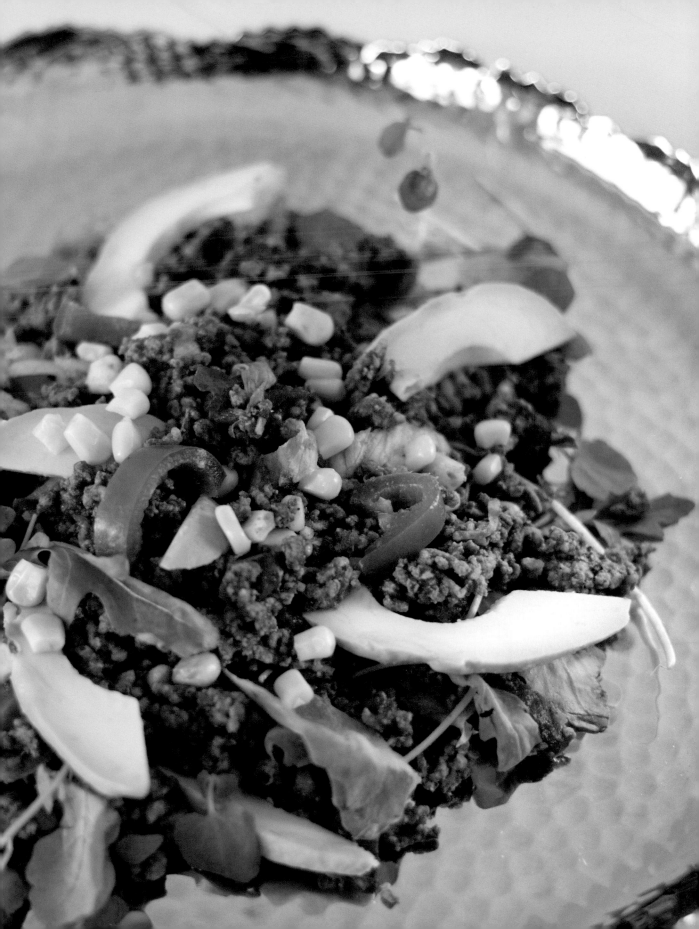

Sushi Salad

I love sushi – and everything Japanese. Most of all, I like the Japanese life expectancy: 86 years for Japanese women, compared to 81 for Irish women! One reason for this is the high consumption of omega-3 fatty acids in the Japanese diet. However, even though the Japanese diet is healthy, you must watch your portions! Rice and oily fish can be high in calories and, without realising, you can pile on the pounds by eating sushi. In this recipe I have given only small portions of rice and fish – but it is enough. Another lesson in portion control! **Serves 2**

FOR THE SUSHI RICE
40g sushi rice
½ tsp rice vinegar
¼ tsp salt

FOR THE SALAD
100g baby leaves and herbs (I use a mix of Asian leaves, rocket, baby spinach, coriander, basil and watercress)
60g sushi-quality salmon or tuna (or 60g smoked salmon), thinly sliced
3 mushrooms (button or shitake), finely sliced
1 red pepper, finely sliced
½ ripe avocado, peeled and finely sliced
2 tbsp beansprouts
¼ chilli, deseeded and finely sliced (optional)

FOR THE DRESSING
20g pickled ginger
2 tsp soy sauce
2–4g wasabi

Cook the rice according to the instructions on the package. When cooked, stir in the rice vinegar and salt. Divide the sushi rice into two portions, shaping each portion into a log shape. Place one log on each serving plate while you prepare the salad.

Combine all of the salad ingredients in a large serving bowl. Combine all of the ingredients for the dressing in a jar with a lid and shake to combine. Drizzle the dressing over the salad and mix well. Arrange the salad on the serving plates with the sushi rice.

APPROXIMATELY 255 KCAL, 4.9G FIBRE AND 9.3g PROTEIN PER SERVING

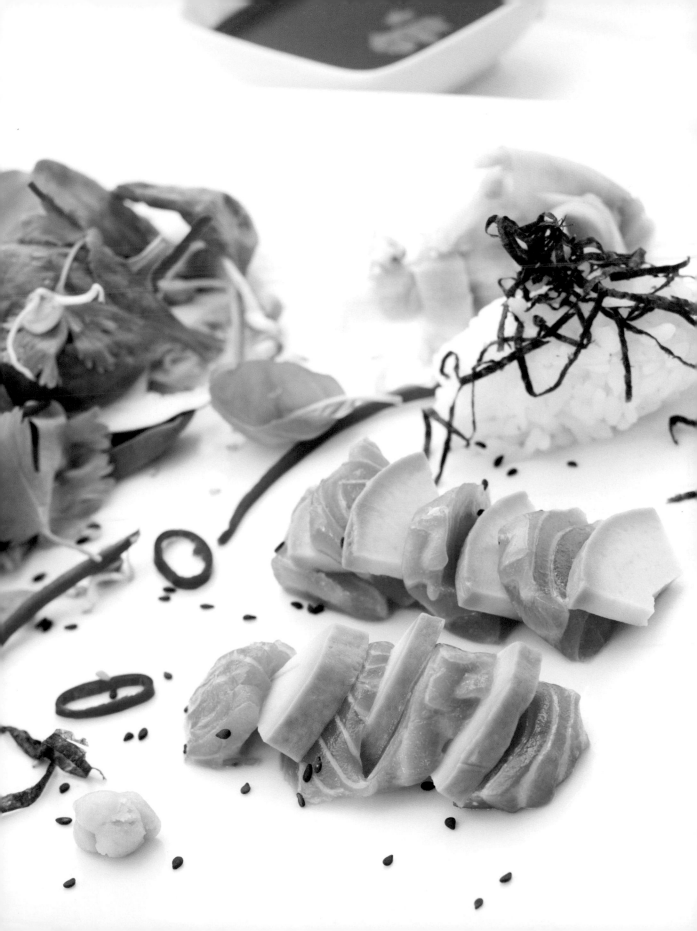

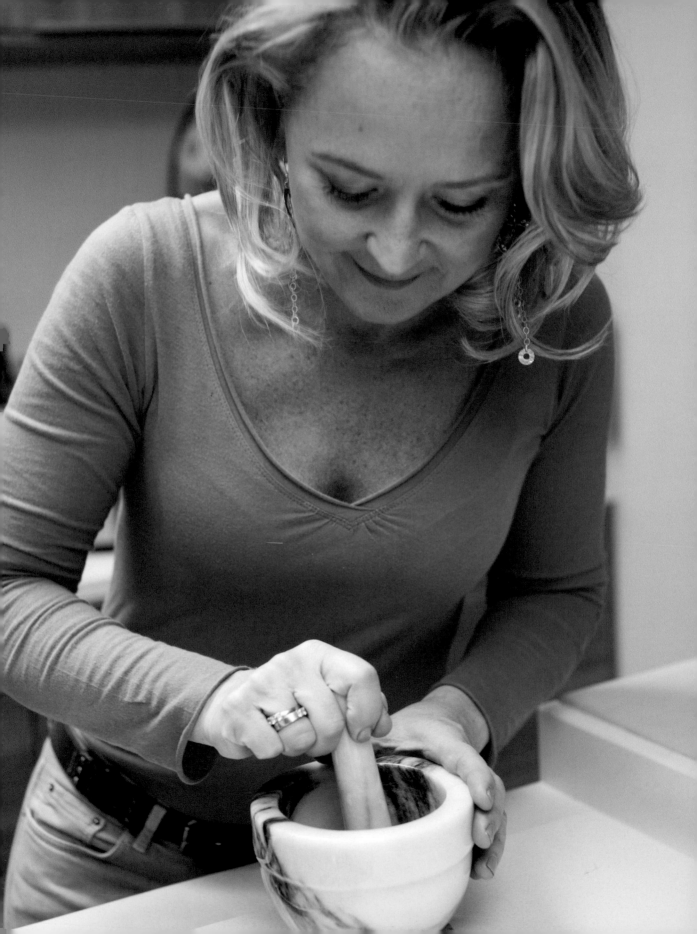

Seafood Salad

For this salad, you will need seafood sticks. They are made from surimi and can be found in large supermarkets or Asian food shops.

This salad dressing is great, and the recipe makes more than you actually need. So use the leftovers on salads and vegetables during the week.

If you can spare some calories and don't have to worry about salt, light feta cheese goes perfectly with these ingredients. **Serves 4**

FOR THE DRESSING
2 egg yolks
2 tbsp white wine vinegar
1 garlic clove, crushed
2 tbsp orange juice
1–2 tsp mustard
1½ tsp ketchup
1 tsp brown sauce
4 tbsp rapeseed oil

2 baby gem lettuce, sliced thinly
200g frozen peas, defrosted in boiling
    water and drained
80g rocket leaves
½ cucumber, cubed
16 baby tomatoes, halved
12 silver skin pickled onions
1 small red onion, finely chopped
3 tsp capers, drained and chopped
120g tin of crabmeat, drained
65g tin of smoked mussels, drained and
    chopped
65g tin of smoked oysters, drained and
    chopped
8 seafood sticks, finely chopped
1 ripe avocado, peeled and quartered
2 hard-boiled eggs, peeled and halved

For the dressing, combine the egg yolks, vinegar, garlic, orange juice, mustard, ketchup and brown sauce in a food processor and pulse a few times to blend. Turn the processor on to a low setting and, with the motor running, add the rapeseed oil in a thin, steady stream through the top of the lid, until you have a thick and creamy dressing.

For the salad, place the lettuce, peas, rocket, cucumber, tomatoes, pickled onions, red onion, capers, crabmeat, mussels, oysters and seafood sticks in a large bowl and mix well to combine.

Divide the salad between four serving plates. Garnish each one with an avocado quarter, half a hard-boiled egg and 2 tablespoons of the dressing.

APPROXIMATELY 350 KCAL, 7.1G FIBRE AND 19.1G PROTEIN PER SERVING

Dinner

My favourite part of the day is when I finally sit down to eat my dinner. Sometimes this is at 6pm – but more often than I'd like, I find myself finishing the last bite at 8pm. This is not the end of the world if you are going to bed around 11pm. But if you like an early bedtime, then have an early dinner.

It is never good to go to bed too soon after dinner: you will end up rolling around with food in your belly, unable to sleep. That is not very relaxing!

I love cooking and would like to spend hours making my dinners! Obviously the time isn't always there, and that's why I've given you some very quick and easy dinner recipes as well as ones that take a bit more time. Some recipes are real family favourites that freeze well too. I've also included some delicious but surprisingly low-calorie recipes – they are good if you've overindulged or if you feel 'stuck' with your weightloss! You'll be able to use many of these recipes at your dinner parties, where your guests will have no idea that they're taking part in the 10lb Diet!

Cowboy Stew

Are you surprised to see a tin of baked beans in a healthy recipe? They are actually a far better ingredient than a lot of commonly used ready-made dinner sauces. Besides their sweet taste, they are also packed with protein and fibre. **Serves 4**

1 tbsp olive oil
400g lean minced beef (or turkey)
1 green pepper, finely chopped
1 yellow pepper, finely chopped
1 red pepper, finely chopped
400g sweet potatoes, peeled and grated
415g tin of baked beans
160ml low fat coconut milk
2 tbsp mild curry powder
2 tbsp soy sauce
½ tsp red chilli powder

Heat the olive oil in a large pan over a medium heat and fry the meat until browned. Lower the heat, add the peppers and cook gently until they have softened. Add the sweet potatoes, baked beans, coconut milk, curry powder, soy sauce and red chilli powder and stir well. Cover and simmer for about 20 minutes, stirring occasionally, until the vegetables are cooked through. Ladle the stew into warmed serving bowls.

APPROXIMATELY 475 KCAL, 11.4G FIBRE AND 29.4G PROTEIN PER SERVING

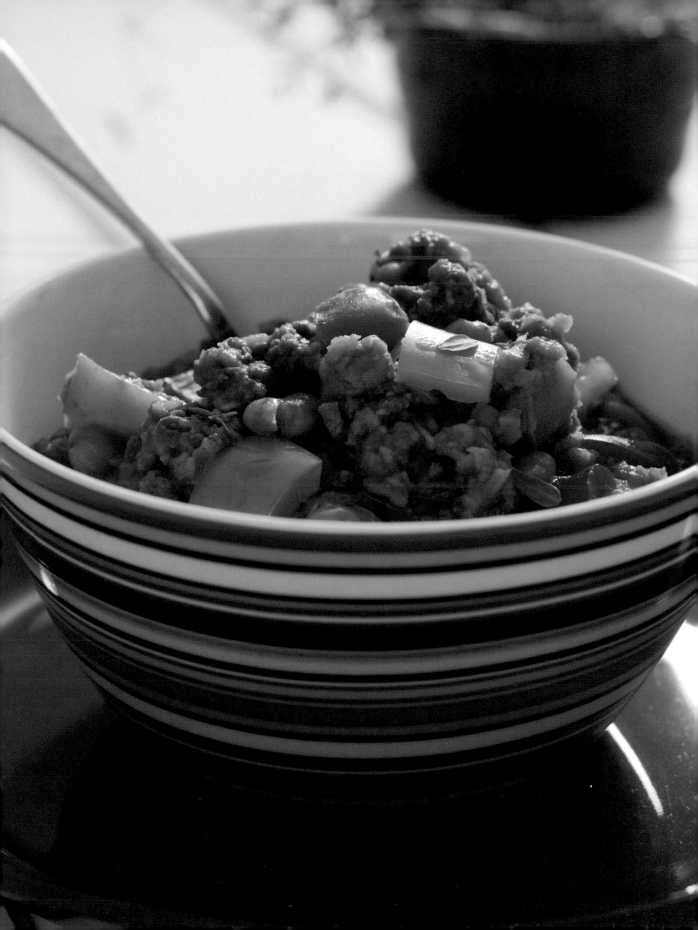

Pomegranate and Beef Casserole

You'll find the pomegranate molasses in any shop that sells Middle Eastern cooking ingredients. Traditionally it is used in casseroles, stews and sauces. It is an ingredient I use in many recipes, so it is well worth searching for. It adds a beautiful, tangy sweetness to dishes. **Serves 4**

1 tbsp olive oil
600g lean stewing beef, cubed
200g shallots, finely chopped
½ celeriac, peeled and diced
200ml beef stock
3 bay leaves
1 tsp black peppercorns
1 red pepper, finely chopped
1 yellow pepper, finely chopped
2 large courgettes, diced
2 celery sticks, finely chopped
20 cherry tomatoes, halved
3 tbsp pomegranate molasses
3 tbsp teriyaki sauce
50g sultanas
Salt and freshly ground black pepper
Seeds from 1 large pomegranate
  (optional)

Preheat the oven to 160°C/325°F/gas 3.

Heat the olive oil in a large casserole over a medium heat and fry the beef until browned on all sides (you may need to do this in batches). Remove with a slotted spoon and set aside.

Add the shallots and fry for 3–5 minutes. Return the beef to the pan. Add the celeriac, stock, bay leaves and peppercorns and stir well.

Add the peppers, courgettes, celery and tomatoes. Stir in the pomegranate molasses, teriyaki sauce and sultanas. Cover the casserole and place in the oven for about 2 hours.

Check the seasoning, then ladle the stew into warmed serving bowls. Sprinkle the pomegranate seeds on top and serve.

APPROXIMATELY 398 KCAL, 7.7G FIBRE AND 41.3G PROTEIN PER SERVING

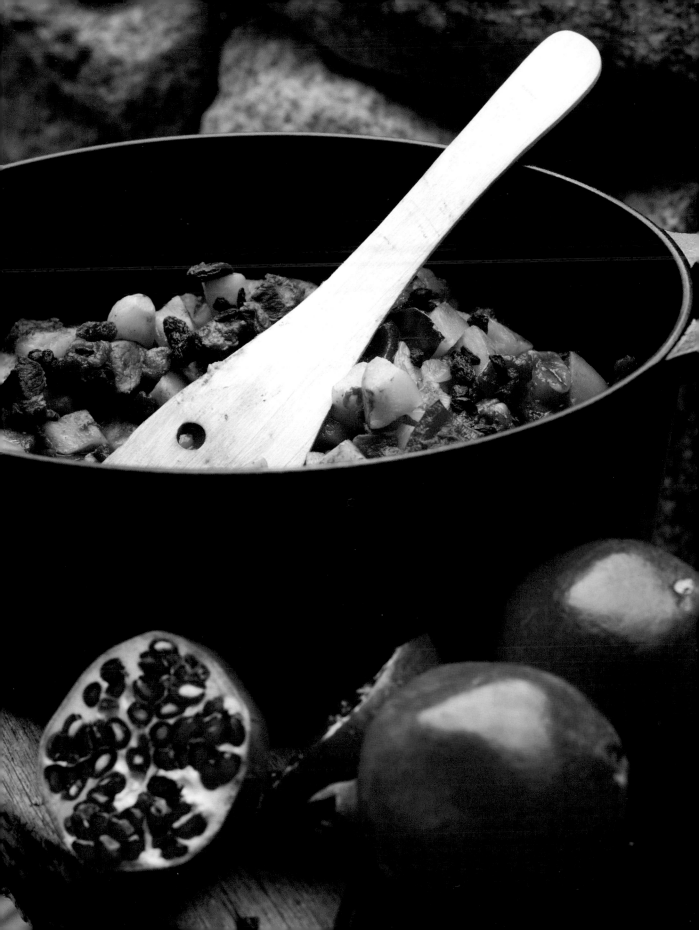

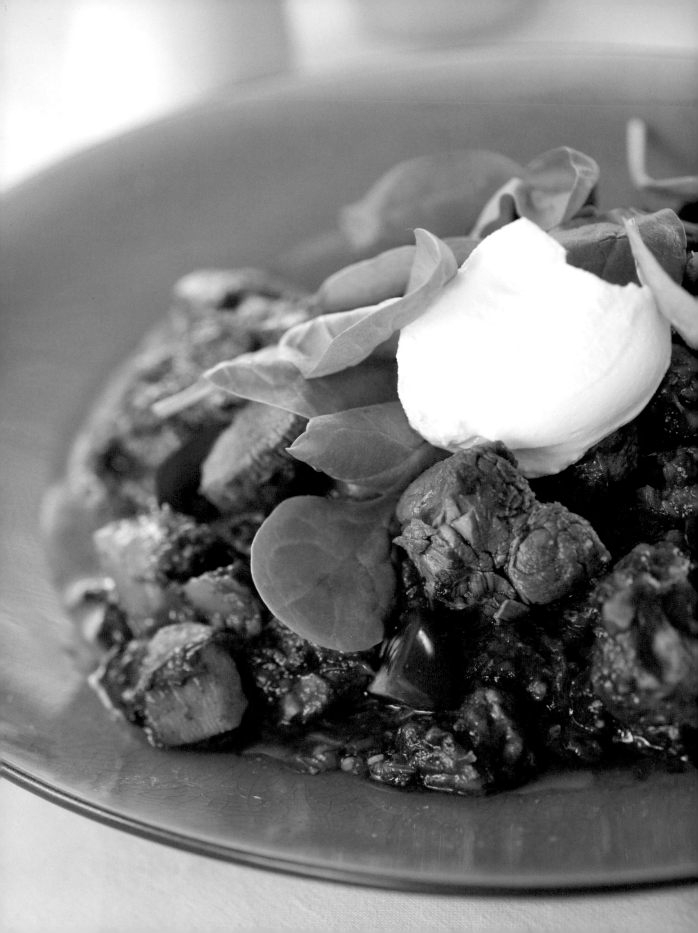

Lamb Rogan Josh

People have a preconception that Indian food is calorific and fatty, since that is what we often get with our typical takeaway. But Indian food can be very healthy and it is thought that the spices used in Indian cooking might have additional health benefits. We now know that turmeric, for example, not only gives food that lovely yellow colour but it also has strong antioxidant and anti-cancer characteristics.

My Rogan Josh includes lots of vegetable fibre and it is an ideal Sunday dinner. While it's in the oven, you can do your daily exercise routine or go for a brisk walk. When you return, there is a piping hot and aromatic dish waiting for you to enjoy!
Serves 4

FOR THE SPICE MIX
6cm cinnamon stick
6–10 black peppercorns
2 black cardamom pods
4 green cardamom pods
2 tsp fennel seeds
1 tsp salt

4 tbsp rapeseed oil
600g lamb, cut into 3cm pieces (ideally leg of lamb)
2 onions, finely sliced
2 tsp ground coriander
2 tsp ground cumin
1 tsp red chilli powder
1 tsp garam masala
1 tsp turmeric
1 celeriac, peeled and diced
400g baby spinach
1 red pepper, finely chopped
1 yellow pepper, finely chopped
2 x 400g tins of chopped tomatoes
3 tbsp Ginger Garlic Paste (p.195)
2 tbsp soured cream or natural yoghurt, to serve
4 tbsp finely chopped fresh coriander, to serve

Preheat the oven to 160°C/325°F/gas 3.

For the spice mix, grind the cinnamon, peppercorns, cardamom, fennel and salt with a pestle and mortar. Set aside.

Heat the rapeseed oil in a large casserole over a medium heat and fry the lamb until browned on all sides (you may need to do this in batches). Remove with a slotted spoon and set side.

Add the onions and fry for 3–5 minutes, until softened. Remove with a slotted spoon and set aside with the lamb.

Add the spice mix to the pan and stir well. Then add the coriander, cumin, chilli powder, garam masala and turmeric. Cook over a low heat for a few minutes, stirring all the time, until the spices have a rich aromatic flavour.

Return the lamb and onions to the pan and mix well to coat everything with the spices. Add the celeriac, spinach, peppers, tomatoes and Ginger Garlic Paste and stir well. Cover the casserole and place in the oven for 45 minutes, then remove the lid and cook uncovered for a further 45 minutes (90 minutes in total).

Ladle the Rogan Josh into warmed serving bowls and top each one with some soured cream and fresh coriander.

APPROXIMATELY 548 KCAL, 8.9G FIBRE AND 32.6G PROTEIN PER SERVING

Stuffed Onions

This dish sounds tricky but it's not! Just give yourself plenty of time to prepare the onions before stuffing them. I have used Mrs H.S. Ball's fruit chutney – my husband's favourite chutney from South Africa. **Serves 4**

8 onions (each one must be around the size of a tennis ball), unpeeled
600g lean minced beef
2 tbsp chopped fresh sage
2 tbsp chopped fresh parsley
2 tbsp spicy fruit chutney, such as Mrs H.S. Ball's
2 tbsp soy sauce
½ tsp salt
2 tbsp grated Parmesan

Preheat the oven to 180°C/350°F/gas 4.

Cut 1cm off the top of each onion. Put the onion tops aside – you will use them as lids later.

Peel the onions. Use a small sharp knife to carefully remove the centre of each onion, leaving just one thick layer of flesh to hold the onion together. Finely chop the removed onion flesh and set it aside.

Mix the beef, sage, parsley, chutney, soy sauce and salt in a large bowl. Stir in the chopped onion flesh and mix well.

Arrange the onions on an ovenproof dish. Spoon the filling into the onions and finish with a layer of grated Parmesan. Replace the (peeled) onion tops and cover the ovenproof dish with foil. Bake the stuffed onions for 30–40 minutes, until the meat is cooked.

Before serving, remove the foil and place the stuffed onions under a hot grill for a few minutes until browned.

APPROXIMATELY 419 KCAL, 5.1G FIBRE AND 38.5G PROTEIN PER SERVING

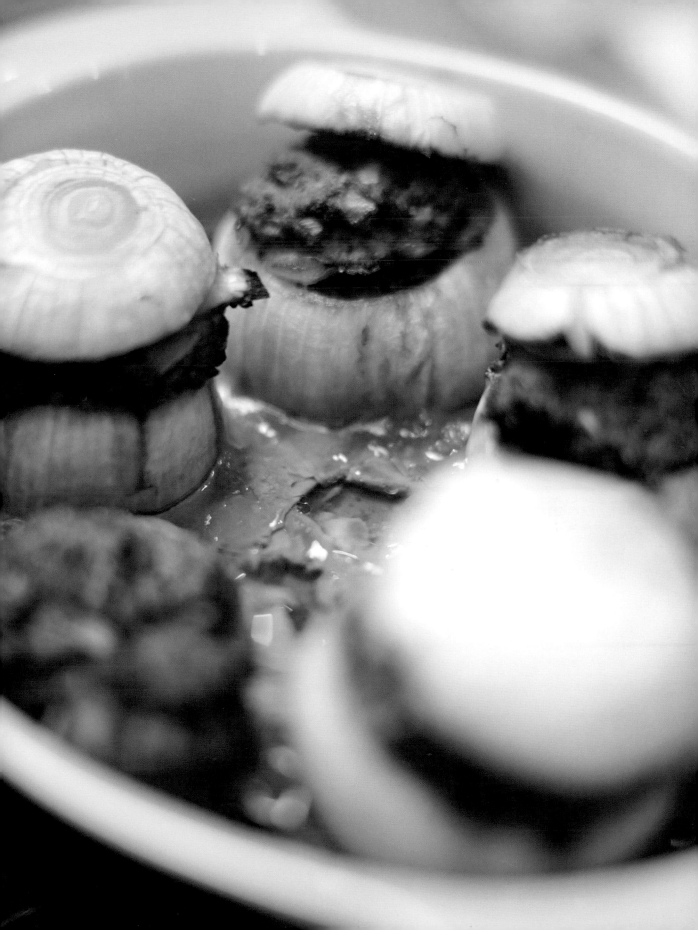

Turkish Pizza

Pizza is one of those foods that is loved by everybody. Italy has a great history of making pizza but so too does Turkey. While pizzas in Italy have tomato sauce, pizzas in Turkey often have tahini instead – and the pizza is topped with tasty minced meat that is cooked in the oven. Even though I love everything Italian, I have to say I prefer the Turkish way of doing pizza.

This pizza has no cheese – and the fresh salad topping is so healthy. Whenever I want to add an extra kick, I mix some crushed garlic with balsamic vinegar and drizzle this over the pizza just before serving. My favourite thing about this pizza is the secret ingredient – sumac. It's tangy and lemony and brings a wonderful Middle Eastern flavour to this pizza. **Serves 4**

FOR THE DOUGH
½ tsp salt
2 tsp (1 x 7g sachet) easy-blend (fast-action) yeast
2 tsp sugar
200ml warm water
2 tbsp olive oil
200g wholegrain spelt flour
150g white flour, plus extra for dusting the work surface

FOR THE TOPPING
400g premium minced beef
1 onion, finely chopped
2 tbsp chopped fresh parsley
2 tbsp pomegranate molasses
1 tbsp sumac
1 tsp cinnamon
1 tsp ground allspice
1 tsp salt
¼ tsp red chilli powder

FOR THE SALAD
90g rocket leaves
1 tomato, chopped
½ cucumber, diced
½ red onion, diced
Salt and black pepper
Juice of ½ lemon

2 tbsp dark tahini paste mixed with 2 tbsp hot water

Make the dough first, since it will need 1 hour to rise. Place the salt, yeast and sugar in a large mixing bowl and stir with a wooden spoon. Pour in the warm water and mix well. Pour in the olive oil and mix well. Now add the flour, a few spoons at a time, mixing well after each addition. It's best to use your hands to mix in the flour. Gradually, it will come together to form a soft dough.

Flour the work surface and turn the dough out onto it. Knead the dough for a few minutes until it is smooth. Shape it into a neat ball, put it back in the mixing bowl and cover the bowl with a damp tea towel. Leave the bowl in a warm, draft-free place for 1 hour, until the dough has nearly doubled in size.

Meanwhile, mix all of the topping ingredients in a large bowl and set aside. Mix all of the salad ingredients in a large bowl and set aside.

When the dough has risen, preheat the oven to 200°C/400°F/gas 6 and dust a large baking sheet with flour. Flour the work surface and knead the dough for a few minutes to knock the air out. Shape the dough into a big circle (or whatever shape will fit your baking sheet). Place the pizza base on the prepared baking sheet.

Use a pastry brush to spread the tahini mixture on the pizza. Arrange the topping evenly on the pizza. Cook the pizza for 12–15 minutes. It is important not to overcook it: you want the dough to be soft around the edges and the meat to be medium-rare.

Cut the cooked pizza into slices, top with the salad and serve without delay.

APPROXIMATELY 570 KCAL, 8.1G FIBRE AND 33.4G PROTEIN PER SERVING

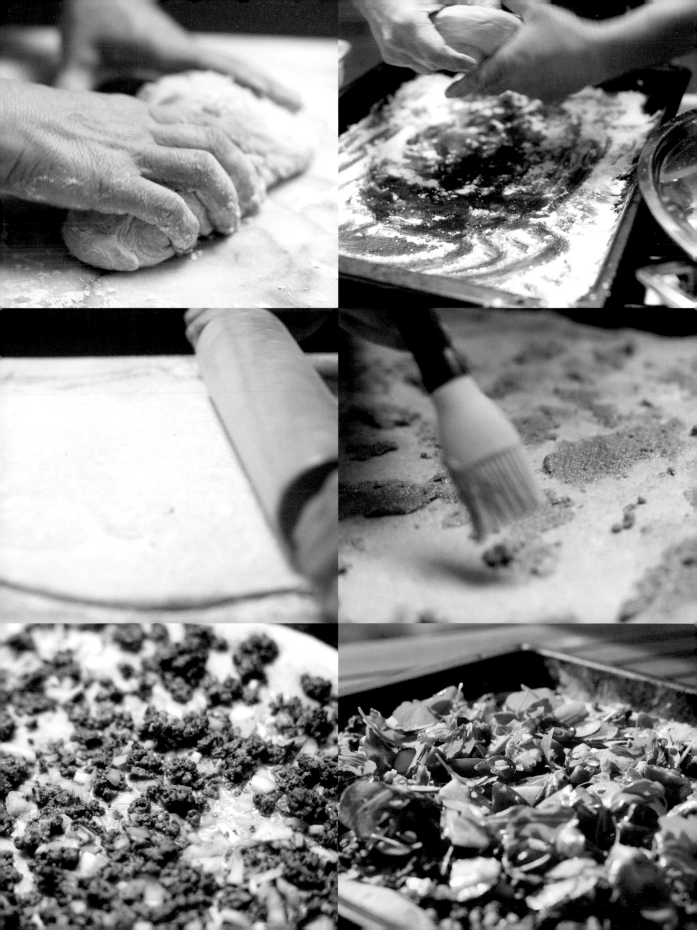

Farmer's Pie

This is a version of shepherd's pie that works well for adults and children alike. I've kept the ingredients very basic. You could probably make this dish the second time around without even needing to see the recipe! **Serves 4**

1 small white cabbage, shredded
200ml beef stock
500g lean minced beef
6 carrots, grated
1 onion, finely chopped
Freshly ground black pepper
6–7 medium potatoes, peeled and quartered
1 tbsp low fat milk
4 low fat Cheddar slices

Preheat the oven to 180°C/350°F/gas 4.

Place the cabbage and stock in a large pan over a medium heat. Cover and simmer for 5 minutes, stirring occasionally. Add the beef, carrots and onion. Season with black pepper and stir well. Cover and simmer for 5 minutes, until the beef turns brown.

Meanwhile, make the mash. Boil the potatoes in salted water for 10–15 minutes until tender. Drain, then mash well with the milk.

Place the cooked mince into an ovenproof dish and top with the mash. Bake for 15 minutes. Then add the cheese slices and bake for another few minutes, until the cheese has melted. Divide the pie between warmed serving bowls.

APPROXIMATELY 515 KCAL, 9.6G FIBRE AND 38.9G PROTEIN PER SERVING

Bacon and Halloumi Stew

This recipe is great for the inexperienced cook, since you cannot really do anything wrong! You can experiment a little with the molasses but bear in mind that it has 50kcal per tablespoon. If you don't like bacon, use turkey rashers – they contain almost the same amount of calories. **Serves 4**

2 tsp butter
100g light halloumi cheese, cubed
4 bacon rashers, rind removed and sliced
1 leek, finely sliced
2 garlic cloves, crushed
½ cabbage (green or white), shredded
2 courgettes, diced
1 red pepper, finely sliced
2 tbsp pomegranate molasses
Freshly ground white pepper

Heat 1 teaspoon of butter in a large pan. Fry the halloumi for a few minutes, until coloured on all sides. Remove from the pan and set aside.

Add the bacon to the pan and cook for 3–5 minutes, stirring frequently. Remove from the pan and set aside with the halloumi.

Add 1 teaspoon of butter to the pan and allow it to melt. Add the leek and garlic and fry for 3 minutes. Add the cabbage and stir well. Reduce the heat and cook, covered, for a few minutes until the cabbage is soft but not soggy.

Add the courgettes and pepper and cook for about 10 minutes to soften the courgette. Return the halloumi and bacon to the pan and reheat gently. Stir in the pomegranate molasses. Season with white pepper and divide the stew between warmed serving bowls.

APPROXIMATELY 186 KCAL, 5.8G FIBRE AND 3.2G PROTEIN PER SERVING

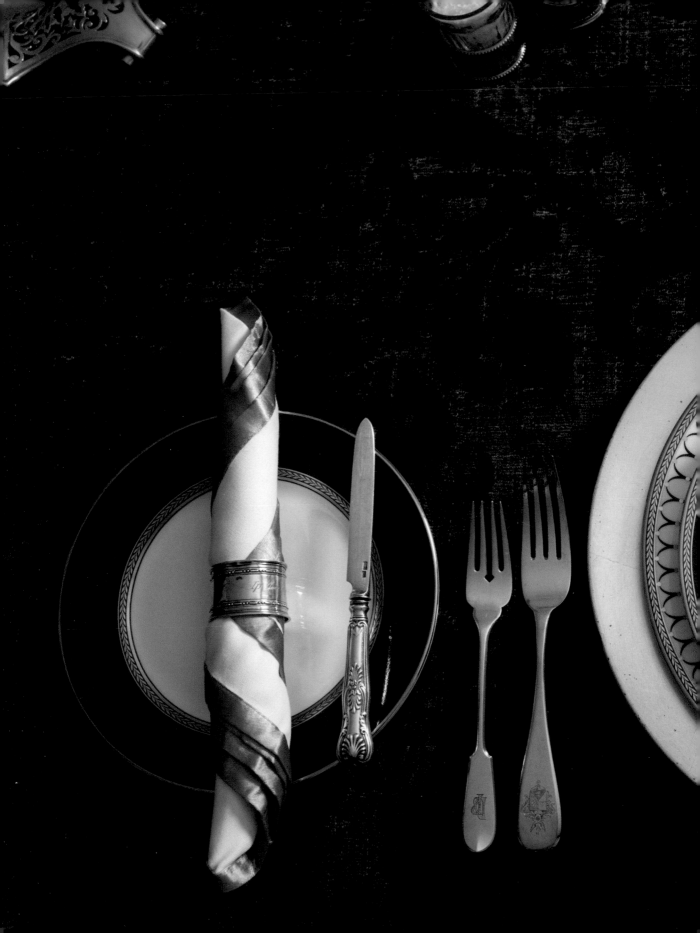

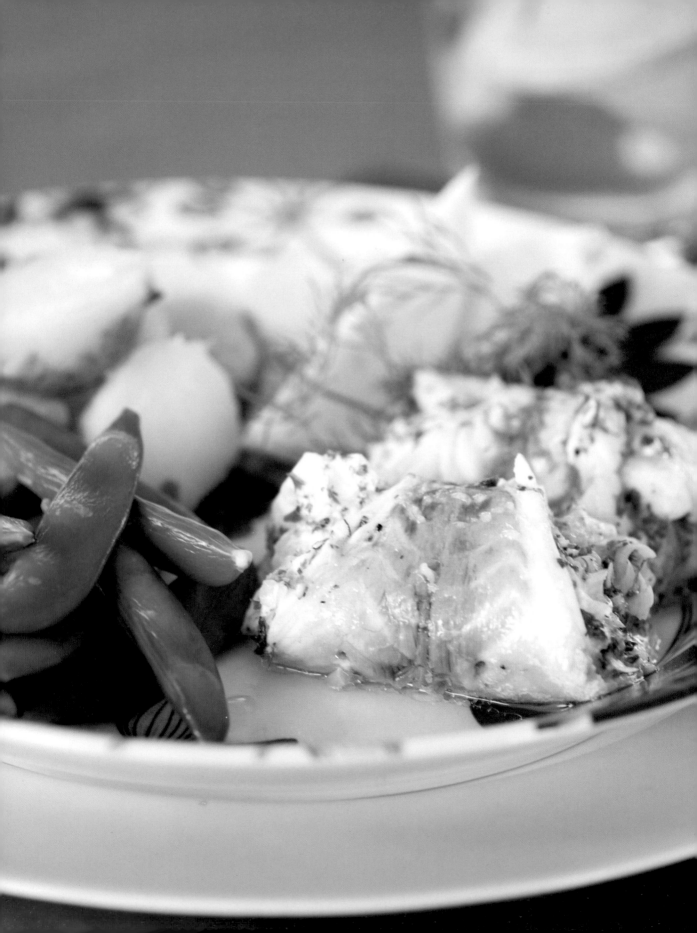

Fish Rolls

I absolutely love this recipe! It is so tasty, yet so simple. You could use herb flavoured cream cheese instead of the fresh herbs, but this dish has a much better flavour if you chop up fresh basil, dill and parsley. I like to serve it with grated carrots and a squeeze of lemon juice. **Serves 4**

100g light soft cheese
4 scallions, finely chopped
1 tbsp chopped fresh basil
1 tbsp chopped fresh dill
1 tbsp chopped fresh parsley
600g hake fillets, skin and pin bones
  removed
Herbamare herbal salt

Combine the cream cheese, scallions, basil, dill and parsley in a medium bowl.

Smear the cheese mixture evenly over the fish fillets. Roll each fillet and secure it with a cocktail stick. Place the fillets in a steamer for 6–8 minutes until cooked through. Season with Herbamare to taste and serve.

APPROXIMATELY 178 KCAL, 0.4G FIBRE AND 31G PROTEIN PER SERVING

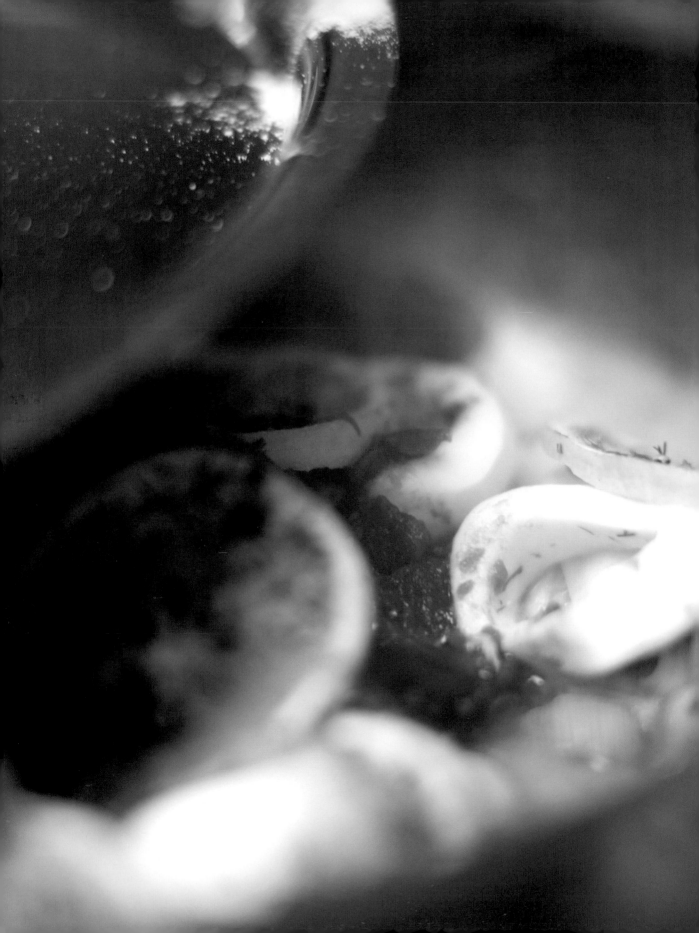

Portuguese Squid

Another tasty and simple fish dinner that goes down a treat in my household! The trick to this recipe is using the freshest ingredients. Try to eat fish three times a week as part of your diet. **Serves 4**

1 tsp butter
4 leeks, sliced into thin rounds
800g squid, cut into 5mm rings
600g fresh plum tomatoes, sliced (or 2 x
    400g tins of whole peeled tomatoes)
Salt and freshly ground black pepper
50g fresh dill, leaves removed and finely
    chopped
1 lemon, sliced

Melt the butter in a large pan over a low heat. Arrange the leeks in a neat layer at the bottom of the pan. Add the squid rings in a neat layer. Arrange the tomato slices on top and season. Sprinkle the dill over the tomatoes and finish with a layer of lemon slices.

Place the pan on a low heat and cook for about 1 hour 30 minutes or until the squid is tender. (The cooking time will be reduced on a gas hob, so check it regularly after the 45-minute mark.) Spoon into warmed serving bowls.

APPROXIMATELY 239 KCAL, 6.0G FIBRE AND 35.3G PROTEIN PER SERVING

Easy Fish Pie

This is such a healthy family dish. If one of the fish varieties used is a smoked fish, like smoked haddock, the flavour is even better. Try to find fish pie mix in your supermarket – it's a selection of fish that's already prepared and ready to go into dishes like this. If you are using fish fillets, make sure they're boneless because it's impossible to pick out bones from a pie like this! **Serves 4**

4 medium potatoes, peeled and quartered
600g frozen leaf spinach, defrosted and drained
2 hard-boiled eggs, peeled and chopped
500g fish pie mix
Fish spice or salt and pepper, for seasoning
1 tbsp olive oil
1 onion, finely chopped
350ml low fat milk
150g low fat cream cheese
100g low fat Cheddar, grated
4 carrots, peeled and cut into thin rounds
400g frozen peas

Preheat the oven to 190°C/375°F/gas 5.

Boil the potatoes in salted water for 10–15 minutes until tender.

Meanwhile, spread the spinach over the base of a deep ovenproof dish. Arrange the hard-boiled eggs and fish pie mix on top of the spinach. Season and set aside.

Heat the olive oil in a large pan over a medium heat and fry the onion for a few minutes, until softened. Add the milk and soft cheese. Cook for 5 minutes, stirring frequently, until smooth. Pour this liquid over the fish in the ovenproof dish, reserving 1 tablespoon to make the mash.

Drain the potatoes and mash them with the reserved liquid. Carefully top the fish mixture with the mashed potatoes. Sprinkle the Cheddar on top of the pie and bake for 25 minutes.

A few minutes before serving, steam the carrots and peas.

Divide the pie between warmed serving plates and serve with the carrots and peas.

APPROXIMATELY 549 KCAL, 12.0G FIBRE AND 49.4G PROTEIN PER SERVING

Creamy Prawn Risotto

This is my lower calorie version of a risotto – the ultimate comfort food. By reducing the quantity of rice and adding the butternut and leeks, I was able to lower the overall calorie content. I've kept the ingredients basic, since that's exactly how risotto should be. **Serves 4**

1 butternut squash, peeled, deseeded and cut into 2cm cubes
1 leek, finely chopped
100g arborio risotto rice
600ml vegetable stock, simmering
200g frozen prawns, thawed, cooked and peeled
50g low fat cream cheese
2 tsp freshly chopped dill, to serve
Juice of ½ lemon, to serve

Place the butternut, leek and rice in a large pan and add just enough water to cover. Heat the pan over a medium heat and bring to the boil, uncovered.

Reduce the heat and add a ladleful of simmering vegetable stock. Stir well to mix and, once absorbed, add another ladleful, stirring frequently. The butternut and rice will take about 20 minutes to cook and, during that time, you should be able to incorporate all of the simmering stock. If you run out of stock, add a little boiled water from the kettle.

When the rice is al dente and the butternut is tender, add the prawns and cream cheese and stir well. Reheat gently, then serve the risotto in warmed serving bowls with a sprinkling of dill and a squeeze of lemon juice.

APPROXIMATELY 233 KCAL, 3.7G FIBRE AND 15.5G PROTEIN PER SERVING

Prawn Stir-Fry

You could easily serve this at a dinner party without anyone thinking of it as a diet dinner. The Konnyaku noodles are a great way to add bulk without adding calories.

Serves 4

1 tbsp Ginger Garlic Paste (p.195)
2 courgettes, finely sliced
2 pak choi, shredded
2 red peppers, finely sliced
1 leek, finely sliced
450g baby spinach
1 tbsp fish sauce
1 tbsp oyster sauce
1 tbsp soy sauce
1 tbsp yellow curry paste
200g beansprouts
80ml coconut milk
600g frozen prawns
Konnyaku noodles, rinsed

Heat the Ginger Garlic Paste in a large pan (or lidded wok) over a medium-high heat and add the courgettes, pak choi, peppers and leek. Stir well, cover and allow the vegetables to cook for about 3 minutes. Add the spinach and stir well. When the spinach begins to wilt, add the fish sauce, oyster sauce, soy sauce and yellow curry paste. Add the beansprouts and coconut milk and stir well. Cover and simmer for 2–3 minutes, or until the vegetables are tender.

Add the frozen prawns: as they cook, they will release enough liquid to make the stir-fry sauce. When the prawns are cooked, stir in the noodles and reheat gently for 2–3 minutes. Divide the stir-fry into warmed bowls and serve without delay.

APPROXIMATELY 310 KCAL, 7.2G FIBRE AND 35.1G PROTEIN PER SERVING

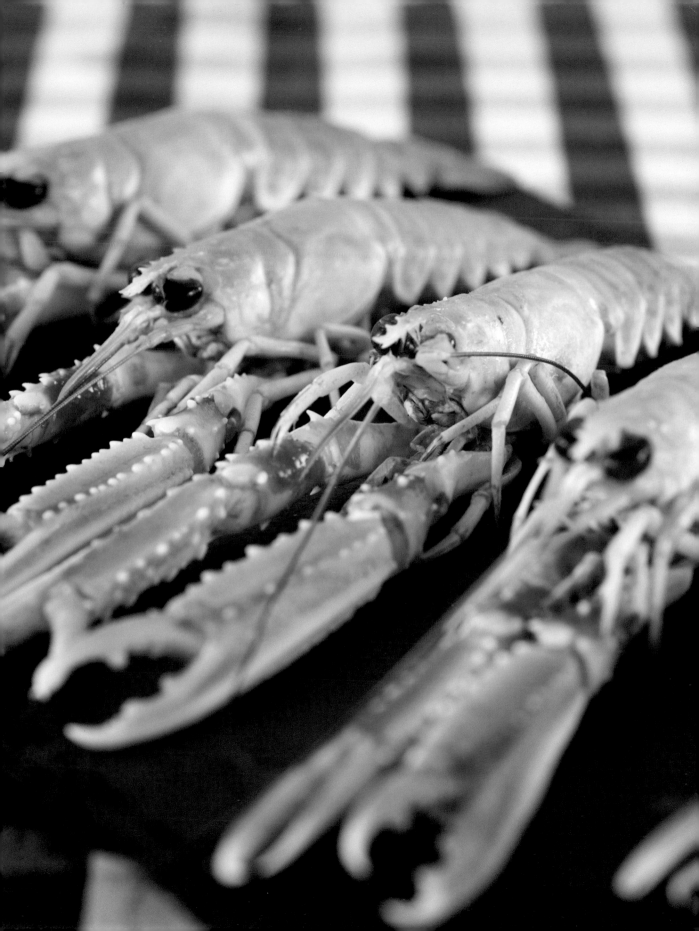

Fish with Mushroom Sauce

Fish is such a healthy ingredient in your diet, since it is both high in protein and low in fat. When you eat low fat protein such as fish, you can well afford to eat something like this mushroom sauce on the side. Of course, the sauce does not have to be eaten with fish – it goes very well with chicken also. **Serves 4**

800g cod or hake fillet, skin and pin
    bones removed
4 carrots, roughly chopped
400g broccoli, broken into florets
1 tsp olive oil
400g mushrooms, finely sliced
2 onions, finely sliced
40ml soy sauce, plus extra to serve
120g low fat cream cheese
200ml low fat milk

Place the fish in a steamer basket. Place the carrots and broccoli in another steamer basket. Cook the fish and vegetables for about 12 minutes, until tender.

Meanwhile, heat the olive oil in a large pan over a medium heat. Add the mushrooms, onions, soy sauce, cream cheese and milk. Stir well to combine the ingredients. Reduce the heat, cover and leave to simmer for 5–10 minutes.

Arrange the cooked fish, carrots and broccoli on warmed serving plates and sprinkle them with a few drops of soy sauce. Spoon the mushroom sauce over the fish and serve.

APPROXIMATELY 368 KCAL, 8.7G FIBRE AND 51.1G PROTEIN PER SERVING

Baked Trout

It is important to have some oily fish in your diet – and trout is very easy to bake in the oven. This dinner is even better with a serving of Cauliflower Mash on the side. **Serves 4**

600g trout fillet, skin and pin bones removed
2 tbsp sweet chilli sauce
400g broccoli, broken into florets
8 carrots, roughly chopped
2 quantities of the Cauliflower Mash on p.184 (optional)

Preheat the oven to 200°C/400°F/gas 6.

Place the trout fillets on a piece of foil and pour the sweet chilli sauce evenly over the fillets. Seal the foil and place the trout on an ovenproof dish. Bake for about 20 minutes.

Meanwhile, cook the broccoli and carrots in a steamer until tender.

Divide the cooked trout and vegetables between warmed serving plates and serve with the Cauliflower Mash.

APPROXIMATELY 294 KCAL, 6.0G FIBRE AND 36.1G PROTEIN PER SERVING

Turkey Burgers with Celeriac Chips

Burger and chips – on a diet? Yes, you've read it right! The celeriac chips get a fantastic colour from the turmeric, making them look more like fried chips. I believe this kind of recipe makes a diet feel a lot less negative! **Serves 4**

FOR THE CHIPS
1 teaspoon rapeseed oil
1 teaspoon turmeric
1 celeriac, peeled and cut into medium chips

Cooking spray
4 x 120g turkey breasts, flattened with meat tenderiser
Coarse sea salt
4 mini burger buns
100g lettuce, shredded
1 cucumber, sliced
2 tomatoes, sliced

Preheat the oven to 180°C/350°F/gas 4.

For the chips, mix the oil and turmeric in a large bowl. Toss in the celeriac chips and mix well with your hands to give the chips an even coating of oil. Spread the chips on a baking sheet and roast for about 30 minutes.

About 10 minutes before the chips are ready, prepare the turkey burgers. Lightly spray a wide non-stick pan with cooking spray and place it over a medium heat. Sprinkle a little sea salt on both sides of each turkey breast. Fry the breasts for 2–3 minutes on each side, until cooked through.

Layer the turkey, lettuce, cucumber and tomato on the burger buns and serve with the celeriac chips.

APPROXIMATELY 315 KCAL, 5.2G FIBRE AND 37.0G PROTEIN PER SERVING

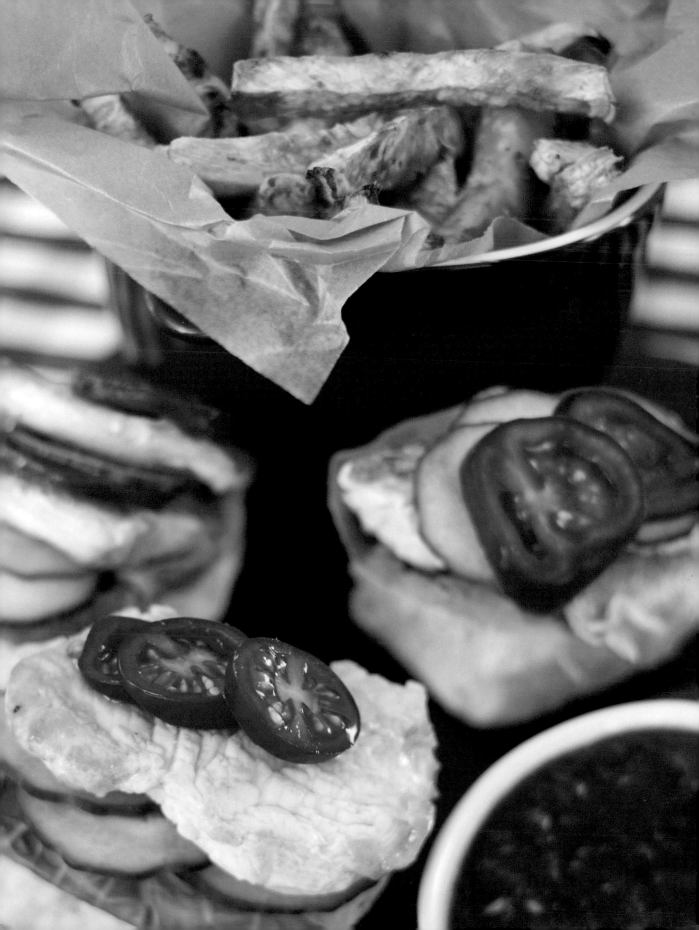

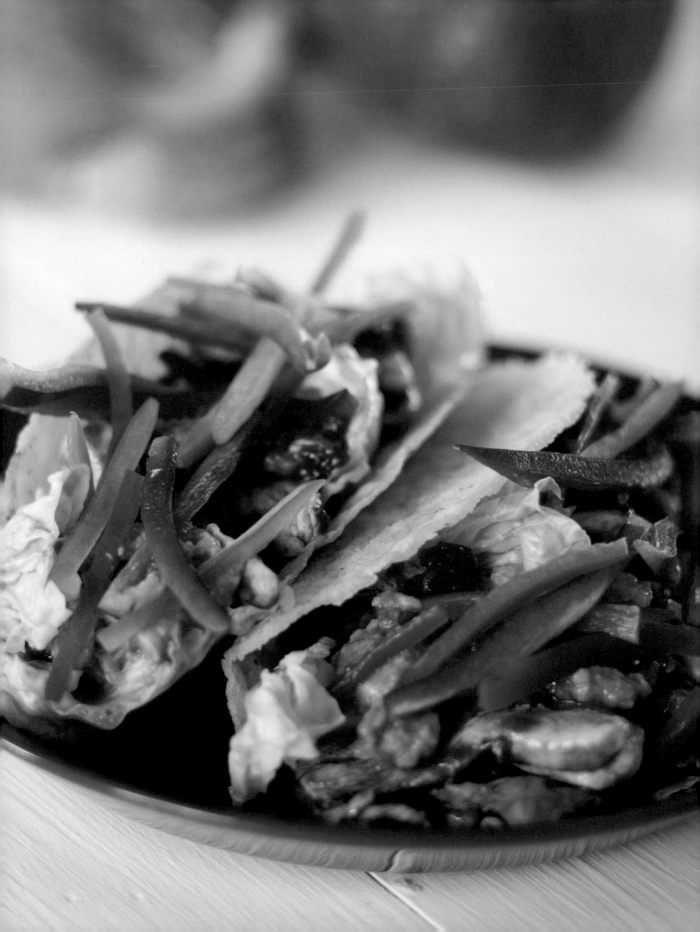

Spicy Chicken Tacos

This is a real Saturday night treat. Guacamole is best when it's made fresh, but get your avocados ready a few days before and ripen them at home. Use some of the salsa from my Tex-Mex Salad (p.98) to increase the heat, or just add a few jalapeños if you like! **Serves 4**

FOR THE GUACAMOLE
1 ripe avocado, peeled and cubed
½ onion, peeled and chopped
2 tbsp whole peeled tomatoes
Juice of ½ lemon
Salt and freshly ground black pepper
½ tsp red chilli powder (if you want a little bit of a kick!)

1 tsp olive oil
4 skinless chicken breast fillets, sliced into medium strips
1 red chilli, deseeded and finely sliced
½ can of whole peeled tomatoes (plus 2 tbsp extra for the guacamole)
Salt and freshly ground black pepper
170g baby gem lettuce, shredded
1 red pepper, finely sliced
1 yellow pepper, finely sliced
1 green pepper, finely sliced
8 ready-made taco shells, warmed

Place all of the ingredients for the guacamole in a food processor and blend until smooth. Scoop the guacamole into a serving bowl and set aside.

Heat the oil in a non-stick frying pan over a medium heat. Fry the chicken until just cooked. Add the chilli, tomatoes, ½ teaspoon salt and a little black pepper and stir well. Reduce the heat and keep the sauce warm while you prepare to serve.

Arrange the lettuce and peppers on a serving platter with the bowl of guacamole. Spoon the chicken and sauce into the taco shells and place on the serving platter.

APPROXIMATELY 447 KCAL, 5.8G FIBRE AND 35.3G PROTEIN PER SERVING

Chicken Fried Rice

If you cook the rice the day before, then this recipe is nearly there. But it's not just a great way to use leftover rice – it's really tasty too. **Serves 4**

200g basmati rice, cooked and left to
   go cold
800g broccoli, broken into small florets
2 tbsp rapeseed oil
4 skinless chicken breast fillets, sliced
   into thin strips
2 eggs, lightly beaten
250g frozen peas, cooked and drained
½ tsp salt
Freshly ground black pepper

Cook the broccoli in a steamer for 10 minutes, or until tender. Drain and keep warm.

Meanwhile, heat 1 tablespoon of rapeseed oil in a wide, deep non-stick pan over a medium heat. Fry the chicken strips until just cooked. Remove from the pan and set aside.

Add the remaining rapeseed oil to the pan. Increase the heat and allow the oil to become quite hot. Pour in the eggs and use a spatula to move them around the pan until cooked. Add in the cooked rice, peas and chicken strips. Stir well and reheat thoroughly. Season to taste. Spoon the rice into warmed bowls and serve with the broccoli.

APPROXIMATELY 481 KCAL, 9.7G FIBRE AND 42.6G PROTEIN PER SERVING

Turkey Meatballs in Tomato Sauce

This method of cooking the meatballs in the sauce saves both time and calories. It leaves them wonderfully moist too! You need to use a saucepan wide enough to fit the meatballs side by side, so be prepared. **Serves 4**

FOR THE TURKEY MEATBALLS
1 tsp olive oil
1 leek, finely chopped
4 garlic cloves, crushed
500g minced turkey
1 tbsp freshly chopped coriander
1 tsp ground cumin
Freshly ground white pepper

1 tablespoon olive oil
1 leek, finely chopped
½ tsp ground cumin
5 courgettes, finely chopped
400g tin of chopped tomatoes
200g baby spinach
1 tbsp soy sauce
Chilli powder
200g spaghetti
50g low fat cream cheese

To prepare the meatballs, heat 1 teaspoon of olive oil in a small pan over a medium heat. Fry the leek and garlic for about 5 minutes until soft. Allow to cool.

Combine the turkey mince, coriander, cumin and a few grinds of white pepper in a large bowl. Add the cooked leek and garlic and mix well. Using wet hands, roll the mixture into 20 small meatballs.

Now prepare the tomato sauce. Heat 1 tablespoon of olive oil in a large pan over a medium heat. Add the leek, cumin and a few grinds of white pepper and fry gently for a few minutes, until the leek is soft. Stir in the courgettes, tomatoes, spinach, soy sauce and a pinch of chilli powder and mix well.

When the sauce begins to bubble, reduce the heat and add the turkey meatballs one by one. Cook uncovered for about 20 minutes, turning the meatballs occasionally and ladling the sauce over them to keep them moist.

In the meantime, cook the spaghetti according to the instructions on the package.

Just before serving, stir the cream cheese into the sauce and reheat gently. Serve the spaghetti, meatballs and sauce in warmed serving bowls.

APPROXIMATELY 489 KCAL, 6.8G FIBRE AND 47.7G PROTEIN PER SERVING

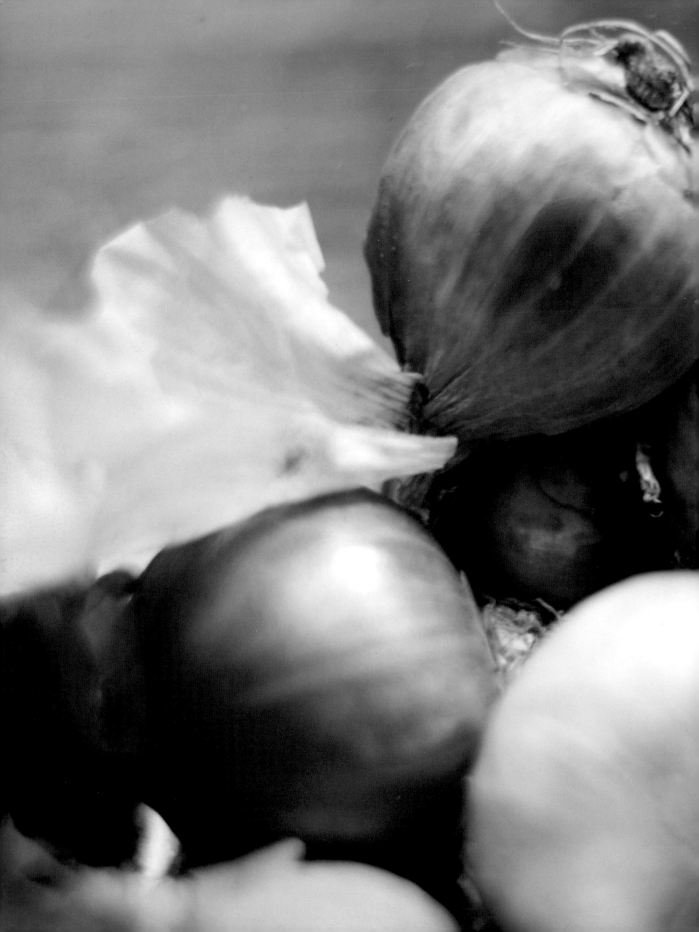

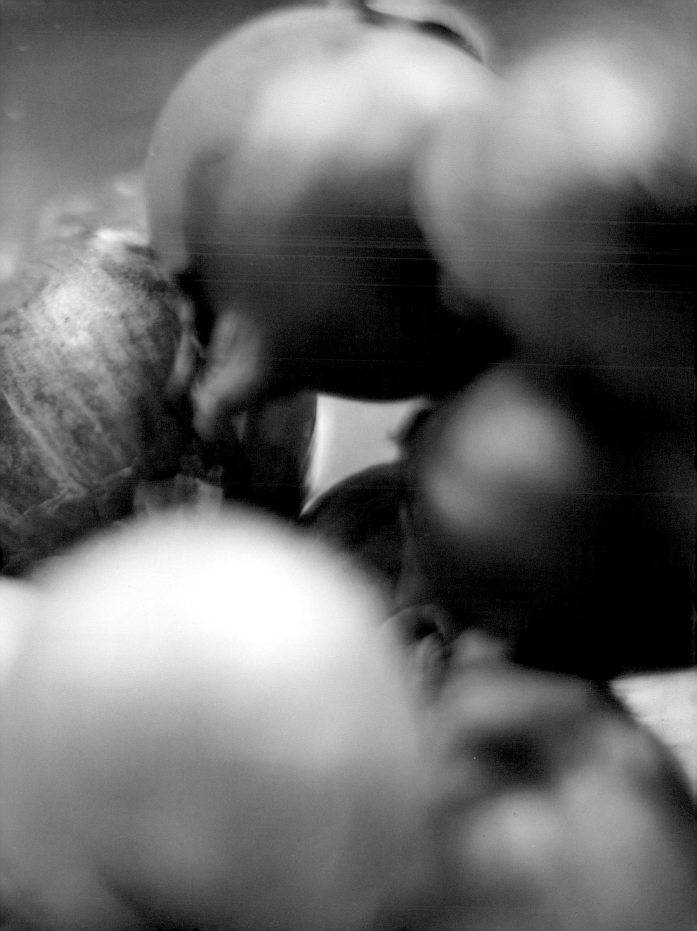

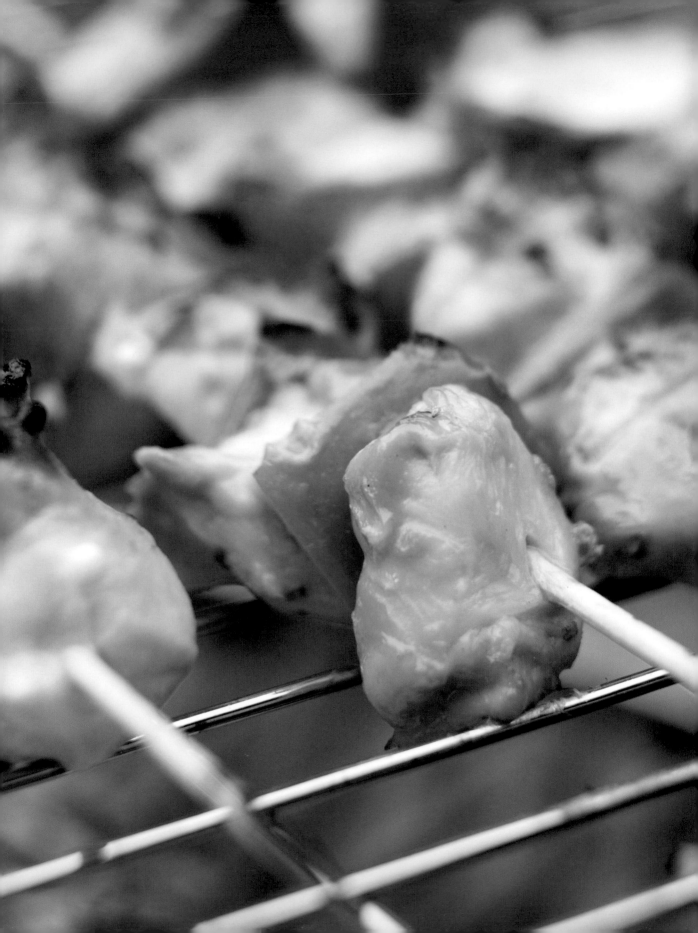

Chicken Kebabs with Pomegranate Molasses

Pomegranate molasses is my secret ingredient for marinades. It gives these kebabs their tangy flavour and helps to tenderise the meat.

You will need to marinate the kebabs for at least a few hours. It's best to be organised and to do this the night before. You can also soak the bamboo skewers in cold water overnight – then you will be sure they won't catch fire on the grill!

Since the calories are quite low in this dish, feel free to bulk it up with a side dish of your choice. **Serves 6 (Makes 12 kebabs)**

FOR THE MARINADE
5 garlic cloves, crushed
2 red or green chillies, deseeded and
   finely chopped
4 tbsp low fat natural yoghurt
1 tbsp olive oil
3 tsp pomegranate molasses
1 tsp finely chopped fresh rosemary
1 tsp soy sauce
1 tsp stevia

6 skinless chicken breast fillets, cut into
   2cm cubes
4 small courgettes, cut into 2cm rounds
1 green pepper, cut into 2cm cubes
1 yellow pepper, cut into 2cm cubes

12 bamboo skewers, soaked in water for
   at least 1 hour

Mix all of the ingredients for the marinade in a large, shallow dish.

On one of the skewers, thread on the ingredients in this order: chicken, green pepper, courgette, chicken, yellow pepper, green pepper, chicken, courgette, yellow pepper, chicken. Repeat to make 12 kebabs in total.

Place the kebabs in the dish with the marinade and turn them until coated. Cover with cling film and leave to marinate in the fridge for at least 1 hour or preferably overnight.

Barbecue the kebabs over a medium-high heat or cook under the grill for 2–3 minutes on each side. Serve two skewers per person.

APPROXIMATELY 235 KCAL, 1.2G FIBRE AND 32.5G PROTEIN PER SERVING

Chicken Tikka Masala

This recipe is such a healthy alternative to the high calorie version you've probably tasted before. You can also make the cauliflower spicy by seasoning it with some of the same spices that are used in the sauce. **Serves 4**

2 tbsp rapeseed or groundnut oil
4 garlic cloves, crushed
2 leeks, finely sliced
4 cm piece of ginger, peeled and grated
1 tbsp ground coriander
1 tbsp cumin
1 tsp garam masala
1 tsp paprika
1 tsp stevia
1 tsp turmeric
¾ tsp chilli powder
4 skinless chicken breast fillets, cubed
2 tbsp soy sauce
2 tbsp tomato purée
250ml chicken stock
1 small cauliflower, broken into florets
2 tbsp natural yogurt

Heat 1 tablespoon of oil in a large pan over a medium heat and fry the garlic, leeks and ginger for 3–5 minutes, until soft. Lower the heat and add the coriander, cumin, garam masala, paprika, stevia, turmeric and chilli powder. Stir well and cook until the spices release a rich aroma. Then remove from the pan and set aside.

Heat the remaining oil in the pan and fry the chicken until golden on all sides. Return the garlic, leeks, ginger and spices to the pan. Add the soy sauce, tomato purée and chicken stock and stir well. Cover and simmer for 30–40 minutes.

About 15 minutes before serving, cook the cauliflower in a steamer until tender.

Before serving, stir the yoghurt into the curry and reheat gently. Serve the curry on beds of steamed cauliflower in warmed serving bowls.

APPROXIMATELY 327 KCAL, 6.8G FIBRE AND 45.6G PROTEIN PER SERVING

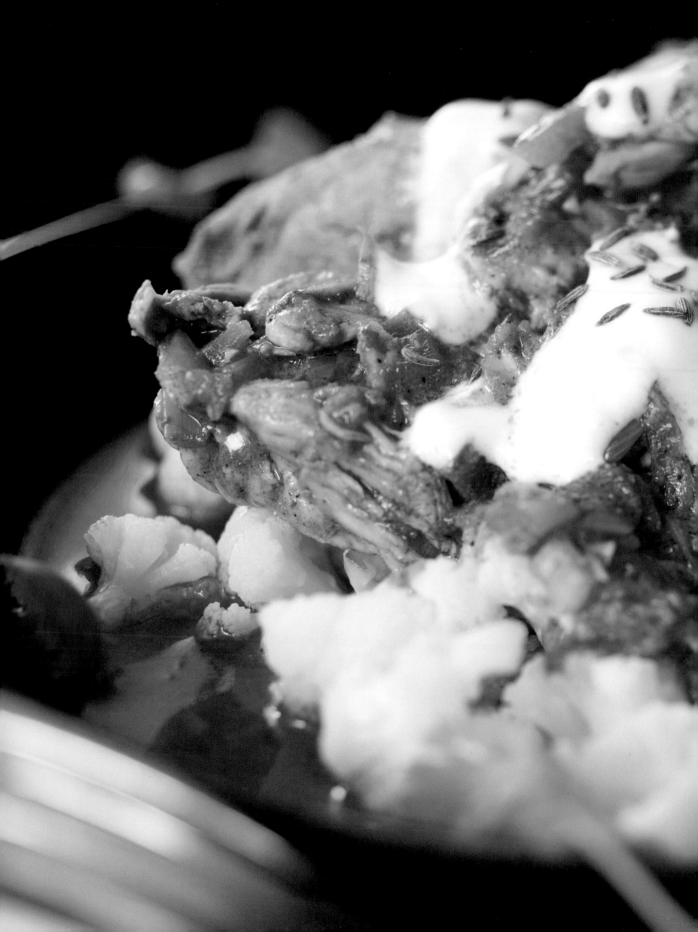

Chicken Butternut Bake

There's something very relaxing about making bakes like this. I like to use a range of colours in the vegetables. I haven't used many spices – on purpose – but feel free to add some if you want. **Serves 4**

Cooking spray
1 large butternut squash, peeled, deseeded and finely sliced
1 carrot, peeled and finely sliced
1 celery stick, finely sliced
1 small onion, finely sliced
4 skinless chicken breast fillets, sliced into thin strips
400g broccoli, broken into small florets
½ 400g tin of chopped tomatoes
1 tbsp soy sauce
1 tsp oregano
50g low fat Cheddar, grated
Salt and freshly ground black pepper

Preheat the oven to 200°C/400°F/gas 4.

Spray the interior of a large ovenproof dish with cooking spray. Layer the butternut slices in the base of the dish. Mix the carrot, celery and onion in a medium bowl, and arrange these vegetables in another layer on top of the butternut. Add a layer of chicken slices and broccoli.

Mix the tomatoes, soy sauce and oregano in a bowl and pour this into the ovenproof dish. Cover the dish with foil and bake in the oven for about 40 minutes. Then remove the foil, sprinkle the Cheddar into the dish and return it to the oven for 5 minutes. Divide the bake between warmed serving bowls. Season and serve.

APPROXIMATELY 347 KCAL, 8.8G FIBRE AND 45.8G PROTEIN PER SERVING

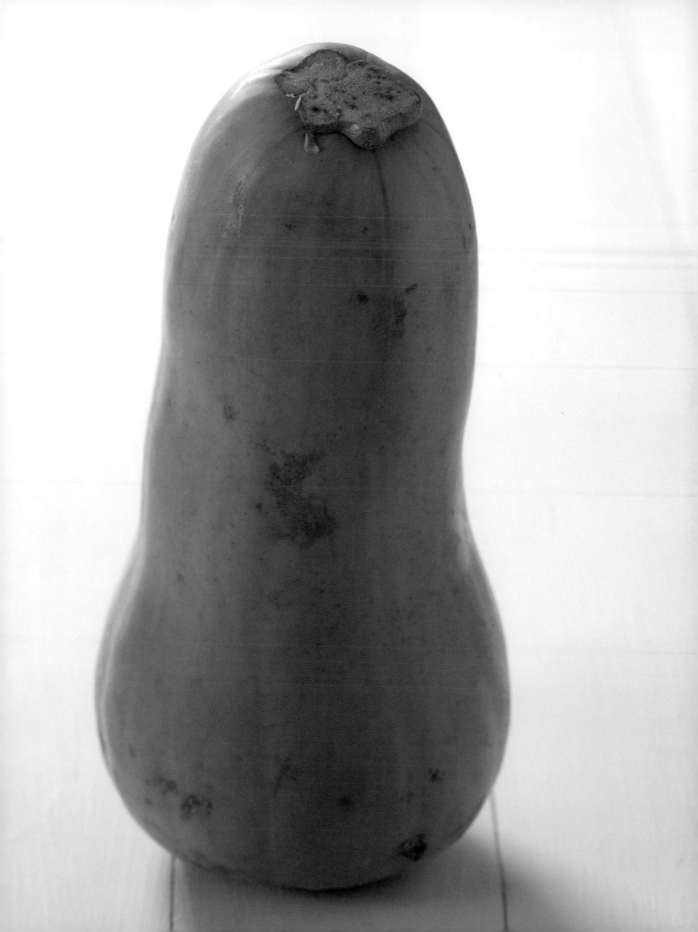

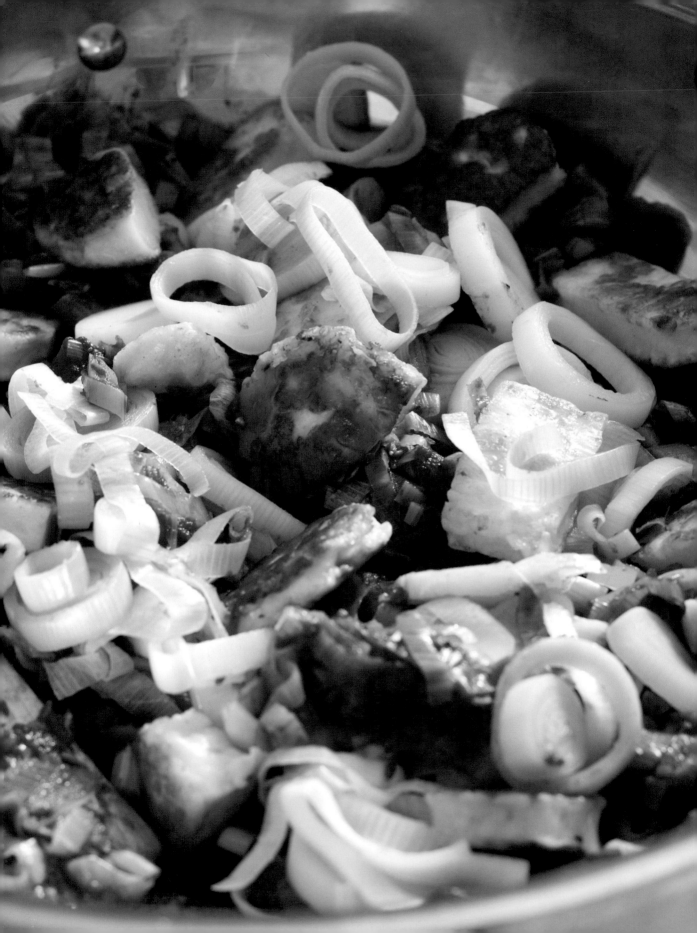

Fried Halloumi and Cumin-Spiced Leeks

Halloumi cheese is one of my favourite cheeses. It's even better when it's fried and its flavour goes particularly well with leeks. Just remember to go easy on the cumin, as too much of it can become overpowering. **Serves 4**

200g brown rice
2 tbsp olive oil
225g low fat halloumi, cubed
2 large leeks, finely sliced
½ tsp ground cumin
Juice of 1 lime
400g tin of chopped tomatoes
Salt
Freshly ground black pepper

Cook the rice according to the instructions on the package.

Meanwhile, heat the oil in a large pan over a medium heat and add the halloumi. Fry the cheese for 1–2 minutes on each side until golden. Using a slotted spoon, remove from the pan, drain on kitchen paper and keep warm while you prepare the spiced leeks.

Add the leeks to the pan and fry for 3–5 minutes, until softened. Add the cumin, lime juice and chopped tomatoes and stir well. Reduce the heat and cook for about 10 minutes. Season to taste. Serve in warmed bowls on a bed of brown rice and top with the fried halloumi.

APPROXIMATELY 359 KCAL, 4.7G FIBRE AND 6.8G PROTEIN PER SERVING

Vegetarian Sausage Stew

It's a good idea to vary your sources of protein between animal protein and vegetarian protein. This way you're likely to get a nice balance of different amino acids. Whether you're a vegetarian or just want a different dish from time to time, this one should keep you nice and full. Use Linda McCartney vegetarian sausages, if you can find them – they are the best! **Serves 4**

4 medium potatoes, peeled and
  quartered
300g broccoli, broken into florets
1 tsp olive oil
1 large onion, finely chopped
8 vegetarian sausages, defrosted and cut
  into small pieces
400g tin of chickpeas, drained
400g tin of chopped tomatoes
100ml vegetable stock
2 tsp balsamic vinegar
2 tbsp finely chopped fresh basil

Cook the potatoes and broccoli in a steamer until tender.

Meanwhile, heat the olive oil in a large pan over a medium heat. Fry the onion and sausage pieces for about 5 minutes. Add the chickpeas, tomatoes, stock, vinegar and 1 tablespoon of basil. Stir well, cover and simmer for 10 minutes.

Divide the steamed potatoes, broccoli and stew between warmed serving bowls and garnish with a sprinkling of chopped basil.

APPROXIMATELY 447 KCAL, 14.3G FIBRE AND 17.7G PROTEIN PER SERVING

Sweet and Sour Stir-Fry

This sweet and sour sauce is made with stevia – I much prefer to use stevia instead of sugar or artificial sweetener. **Serves 4**

FOR THE SWEET AND SOUR SAUCE

2 tbsp cider vinegar

1 tsp ground arrowroot

400g tin of chopped tomatoes, puréed until smooth

1 tbsp soy sauce

1 tbsp stevia

1 tbsp Ginger Garlic Paste (p.195)

4 pak choi, shredded

2 red peppers, finely sliced

2 yellow peppers, finely sliced

1 leek, finely sliced

150g beansprouts

1 tbsp olive oil

400g tofu, patted dry with kitchen towel and cut into cubes

Mix the cider vinegar and arrowroot in a small bowl and set aside for a few minutes, until the paste has doubled in size. Place the puréed tomatoes, soy sauce and stevia in a small pan. Stir in the arrowroot paste and mix well. Simmer for a few minutes, until the sauce is thickened and glistening. Set aside and keep warm.

Heat the Ginger Garlic Paste in a wok or large pan over a medium-high heat. Add all of the vegetables and stir-fry until tender. Remove the cooked vegetables from the pan and keep them warm while you cook the tofu.

Heat the olive oil in the pan. Fry the tofu for 3 minutes on each side, until crispy (you may need to do this in batches).

Return the cooked vegetables to the pan, pour in the sweet and sour sauce and mix well to heat through. Divide the stir-fry between warmed serving bowls. Serve without delay.

APPROXIMATELY 211 KCAL, 6.4G FIBRE AND 12.6G PROTEIN PER SERVING

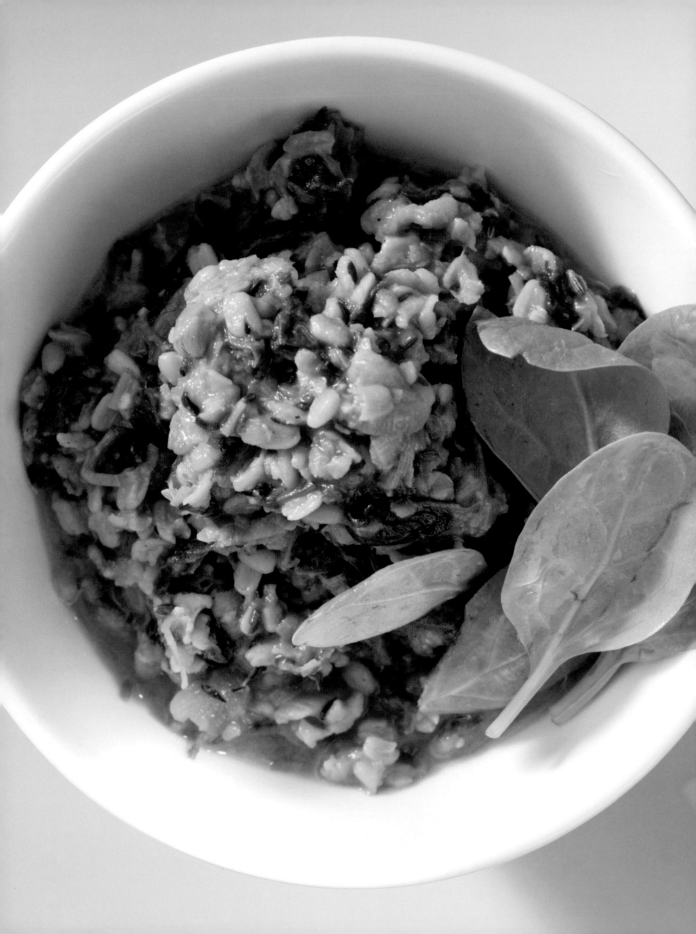

Yellow Dal

So many times I have met vegetarian people who have never cooked lentils! In my opinion, lentils are a cupboard essential – they are just so versatile. If you'd like to include any other vegetables in this dish, just throw them in when you're adding the onion.

You will need to soak the lentils for 6–8 hours. Soaking helps in the absorption of minerals because it breaks the bond of phytates or 'anti-nutrients'. And soaking has another important function: it helps to reduce the flatulent side effects of legumes! **Serves 4**

2 tbsp olive oil
2 tbsp cumin seeds
4 onions, finely chopped
1 large leek, finely chopped
4 garlic cloves, crushed
1 tbsp turmeric
1 tsp chilli powder
1 tsp salt
400g yellow dried split lentils, soaked in water for 6–8 hours, rinsed and drained
300g frozen spinach
200ml light coconut milk

Heat the olive oil in a large pan over a medium heat. Add the cumin seeds and fry for 30 seconds or until they start to crackle. Add the onions and leek and cook until soft. Add the garlic, turmeric, chilli powder, salt and drained lentils and stir well. Add 400ml water, stir well and cover the pot. Simmer for 15 minutes, adding more water as required and stirring well after each addition. (The dal could absorb up to 800ml water.)

When the dal is soft and most of the water has been absorbed, add the frozen spinach. Stir well, cover and simmer until the spinach has defrosted and heated through.

Just before serving, stir in the coconut milk and reheat gently. Divide the dal between warmed serving bowls. Serve as a side dish or add some rice to make a main meal.

APPROXIMATELY 532 KCAL, 17.5G FIBRE AND 29.1G PROTEIN PER SERVING

Vegetable Fajitas

This is a quick but satisfying meal for a busy day. Goats' cheese is a real treat – in this recipe it just melts in your mouth. **Serves 2**

1 tsp olive oil
300g stir-fry vegetables (aubergines, peppers, mushrooms, carrots, onions, scallions, courgettes, broccoli and asparagus work well)
100g tin of black beans, drained
400g tin of chopped tomatoes
2 garlic cloves, crushed
1 tsp finely chopped fresh marjoram
2 wholemeal tortillas
120g goats' cheese

Heat the olive oil in a large pan over a medium heat. Stir-fry the vegetables until tender. Add the black beans, tomatoes, garlic and marjoram and heat through.

Warm the tortillas according to the instructions on the package. Spoon the vegetables and sauce into the tortillas and top with the goats' cheese. Then roll the tortillas and serve on warmed serving plates.

APPROXIMATELY 422 KCAL, 8.3G FIBRE AND 18.3G PROTEIN PER SERVING

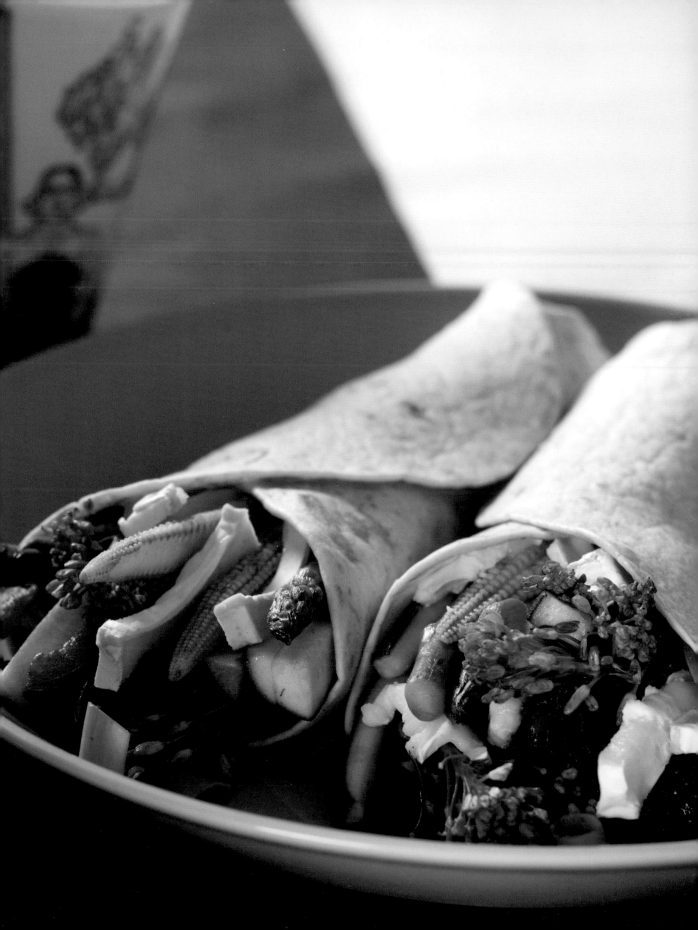

Vegetable Green Curry

This vegetable curry might sound a bit dull but it's actually really tasty – and look at the calories! It goes really well with the Cauliflower Mash (p.184). **Serves 4**

2 aubergines, diced
Salt
1 tbsp coconut oil
2 tsp Thai green curry paste
1 tsp smoked garlic paste
1 leek, finely sliced
½ celeriac, peeled and diced
300ml beef stock
1 tbsp fish sauce
½ red chilli, deseeded and finely chopped
160ml Thai coconut milk (preferably organic)
1 tsp stevia
2 tbsp finely chopped fresh coriander, to serve

Sprinkle the aubergine pieces with salt and leave them to sit in a colander for 15 minutes. Then rinse them under cold water and pat dry.

Meanwhile, heat the coconut oil in a large pan over a medium heat. Add the green curry paste and smoked garlic paste and fry for 1 minute, stirring all the time. Add the leek and celeriac and fry for 3–5 minutes. Add the aubergine, stock, fish sauce and chilli and stir well. Cover and simmer for about 5 minutes.

Stir in the coconut milk and stevia. Cover and simmer for 25 minutes, stirring occasionally. Divide the curry between warmed serving bowls and garnish with coriander.

APPROXIMATELY 172 KCAL, 6.1G FIBRE AND 3.6G PROTEIN PER SERVING

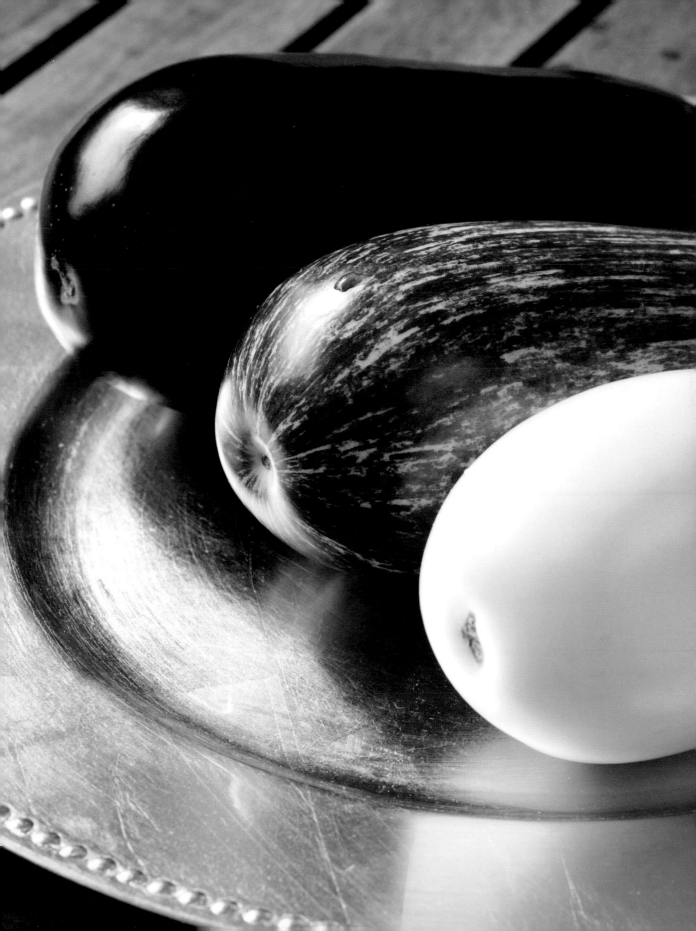

Courgette Bake

This is almost like a vegetarian lasagne without the pasta. Here, the breadcrumbs are the carbohydrate – and they make this dish tasty and crisp. Try it for yourself and see! **Serves 4**

1kg courgettes, finely sliced
Cooking spray
100g Parmesan, grated
200g breadcrumbs
4 eggs, lightly beaten
2 tsp chopped fresh parsley
1 garlic clove, crushed
Salt
Freshly ground white pepper
150g low fat mozzarella, grated

Preheat the oven to 200°C/400°F/gas 6 and line a baking sheet with parchment paper.

Arrange the courgette slices on the baking sheet, spray with cooking spray and bake for 15 minutes.

Meanwhile, combine half of the grated Parmesan with all of the breadcrumbs in a medium bowl and set aside.

Combine the remaining grated Parmesan with the eggs, parsley and garlic in a medium bowl. Season and set aside.

Once the courgette slices are ready, assemble the bake in a large ovenproof dish. Arrange half of the courgettes in a layer on the bottom of the dish. Sprinkle half of the grated mozzarella on top. Add half of the Parmesan breadcrumbs, arranging them in an even layer. Now pour in the egg mixture. Top this with the remaining baked courgettes. Add the remaining Parmesan breadcrumbs, arranging them in an even layer. Finally, top with the remaining grated mozzarella.

Bake in the oven for about 30 minutes, until golden and crispy. Divide the bake between warmed serving bowls.

APPROXIMATELY 424 KCAL, 4.6G FIBRE AND 24.9G PROTEIN PER SERVING

Turnip and Celeriac Bake

Here's a 'shepherd-less pie' for you! The celeriac and turnip work very well together as the mash topping, making this dish lower in carbohydrates than a typical baked pie. This is such a low calorie dish and it's so satisfying. **Serves 4**

Olive oil
½ leek, finely chopped
½ red pepper, finely chopped
2 x 400g tins of chopped tomatoes
250ml beef stock
½ tsp smoked garlic paste

FOR THE MASH
1 celeriac, peeled and cut into 2cm cubes
1 turnip, peeled and cut into 3cm cubes
½ tsp Herbamare herbal salt

Preheat the oven to 180°C/350°F/gas 4. Rub a light coating of olive oil in a large ovenproof dish.

Heat 1 teaspoon of olive oil in a large pan over a low heat. Fry the leek and pepper for a few minutes, until soft. Add the tomatoes, stock and smoked garlic paste and stir well. Leave to simmer, uncovered, for 15–20 minutes until the sauce has thickened.

Meanwhile, make the mash. Cook the celeriac and turnip in a steamer for about 25 minutes until tender. Mash well with the Herbamare.

Pour the tomato sauce into the ovenproof dish. Top with the mash and bake for 15–20 minutes. Divide the bake between warmed serving bowls.

APPROXIMATELY 122 KCAL, 7.7G FIBRE AND 6.0G PROTEIN PER SERVING

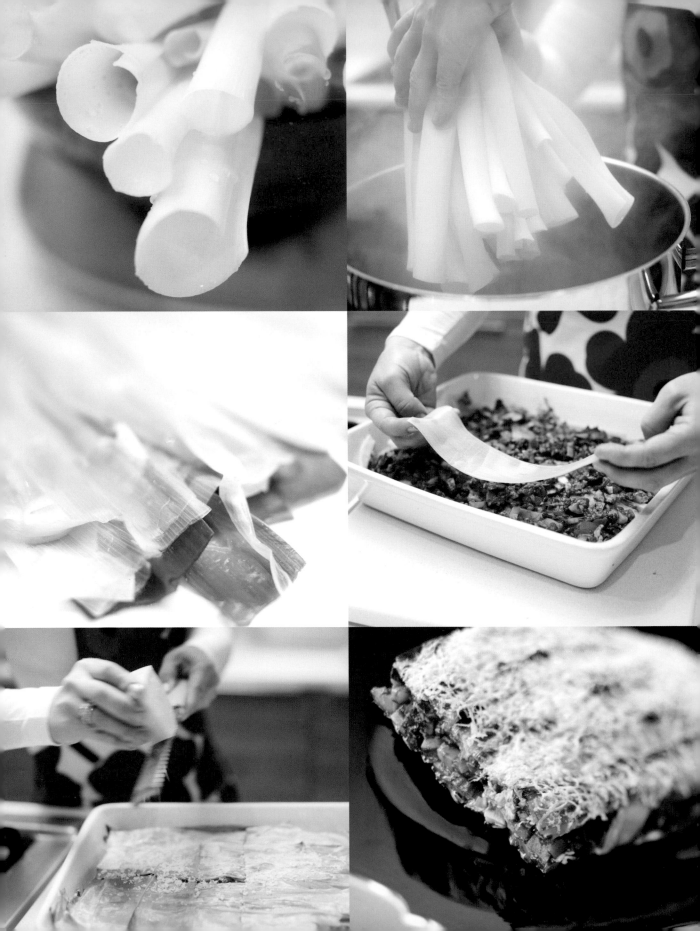

'Now to Wow' Lasagne

Wow – look at the low calorie count of this lasagne! It's a delicious vegetarian dish and it's also gluten-free. The only trick is to find good-quality large leeks that can be used instead of lasagne sheets. If you have any leftover vegetables such as celery or spinach, add them into the sauce. **Serves 4**

7 large leeks
a tsp olive oil
5 courgettes, finely chopped
500g chestnut mushrooms, finely sliced
2 x 400g tins of chopped tomatoes
1 mushroom stock cube, mixed with 2
   tbsp boiling water
1 tbsp smoked garlic paste
Freshly ground black pepper
30g Parmesan, grated

Preheat the oven to 180°C/350°F/gas 4.

Trim the leeks until they are about the same length as your lasagne dish. Boil for 7 minutes, drain and leave until they are cool enough to handle. Carefully cut the leeks lengthways through to the middle but no further. Open the leeks and separate out the larger leaves – these are your lasagne sheets!

Meanwhile, heat 1 teaspoon of olive oil in a large pan over a medium heat. Add the courgettes and mushrooms and fry for about 3 minutes. Stir in the chopped tomatoes, mushroom stock and garlic paste. Leave to simmer, uncovered, until the vegetables are tender. Season to taste.

Rub a light coating of olive oil in a large ovenproof dish. Spoon a layer of the tomato sauce into the dish and top with a layer of leek. Repeat this process, finishing with a layer of leek.

Bake for 30 minutes. Remove from the oven and sprinkle over the Parmesan. Cover with foil and return to the oven for a further 10 minutes. Divide the lasagne into warmed serving bowls.

APPROXIMATELY 212 KCAL, 9.8G FIBRE AND 15.7G PROTEIN PER SERVING

Chilli Pasta Bolognese

This recipe is amazingly low in fat. Choose your favourite pasta for serving. Use fresh chilli instead of powdered – if you're up for it! **Serves 4**

400g minced turkey
2 turkey rashers, sliced
1 large onion, finely chopped
2 celery sticks, diced
4 small courgettes, topped, tailed and grated
2 x 400g tins of whole peeled tomatoes
½ tsp chilli powder
½ tsp paprika
½ tsp salt
200g wholewheat fettuccine, tagliatelle or spaghetti

Heat a large pan over a medium heat (there is no need for oil). Add the turkey mince and rashers and cook until beginning to brown. Add the onion, celery, courgettes, tomatoes, chilli powder, paprika and salt. Stir well and leave to simmer (uncovered) for about 20 minutes.

Meanwhile, cook the pasta according to the instructions on the package.

Divide the cooked pasta between warmed serving bowls. Ladle the Bolognese on top and serve.

APPROXIMATELY 378 KCAL, 8.9G FIBRE AND 36.4G PROTEIN PER SERVING

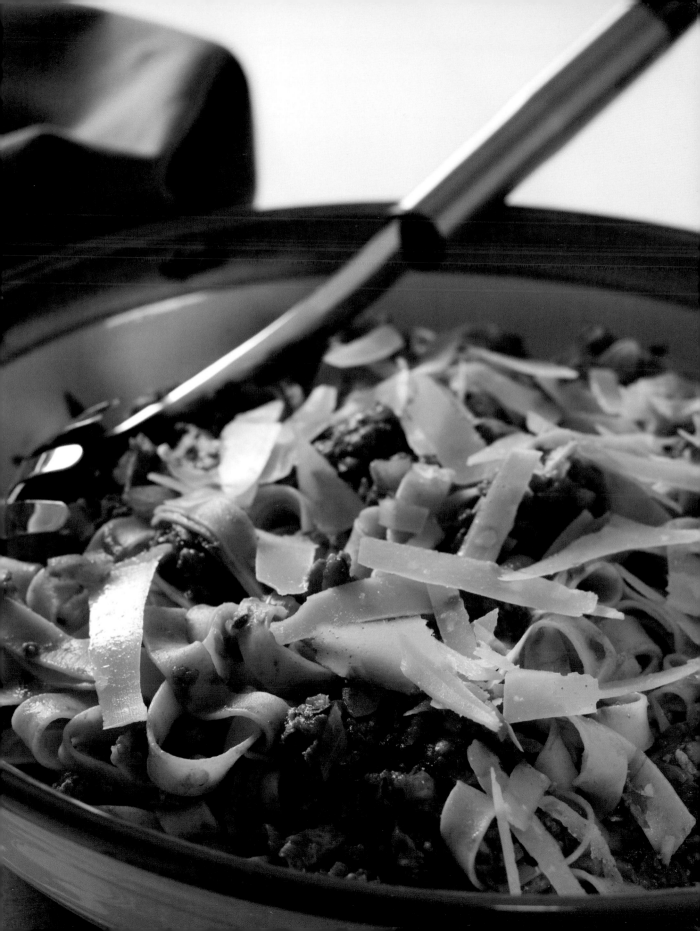

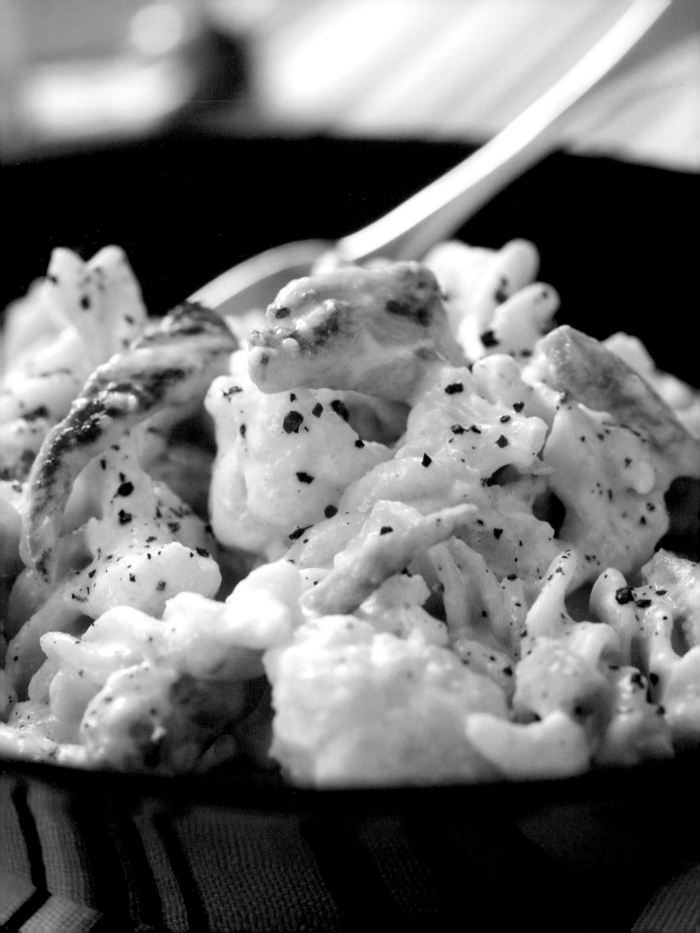

Easy Cauliflower Carbonara

This variety of a classic carbonara works surprisingly well. It is lovely on a cold winter's evening. **Serves 4**

1 tbsp olive oil
200g back bacon, fat removed, diced
2–3 garlic cloves, crushed
200g wholewheat pasta
400g cauliflower, broken into small florets
100g Parmesan, grated

FOR THE SAUCE
2 egg yolks
200ml low fat crème fraîche
50ml low fat milk
Freshly ground black pepper to taste

Heat the olive oil in a medium pan over a medium heat. Fry the bacon and garlic for about 5 minutes and set aside.

Mix all of the ingredients for the sauce and set aside.

Cook the pasta according to the instructions on the package. Halfway through cooking time (about 4 minutes in) add the cauliflower florets and cook them with the pasta.

As soon as the pasta and cauliflower are al dente, drain them and return them to their cooking pan. Add the cooked bacon and garlic and the Parmesan and stir well. Tip in the egg mixture and stir quickly – the mixture will cook on contact with the hot pasta and cauliflower, and it will form a sauce.

Spoon the Carbonara into warmed serving bowls – and get to the dinner table immediately!

APPROXIMATELY 538 KCAL, 8.1G FIBRE AND 33.9G PROTEIN PER SERVING

Creamy Ham and Garlic Pasta

When I lived in Italy, I loved how the people could make a comforting dinner with some pasta and just a few really basic ingredients. This pasta is no-fuss food. I actually cheat a bit by using a ready-made sauce – but it's delicious and the calories aren't too bad at all. **Serves 4**

200g pasta shells
400g frozen peas
100g frozen sweetcorn
200g packet of Philadelphia Simply Stir cooking sauce (I like mushroom flavour)
10 slices of cooked ham (180g), finely chopped

Cook the pasta according to the instructions on the package. About 3 minutes from the end, add the peas and sweetcorn to the pot with the pasta.

Drain the pasta, peas and sweetcorn and return them to the pan. Stir in the Philadelphia cooking sauce and ham. Gently reheat, then divide the pasta between warmed serving bowls.

APPROXIMATELY 365 KCAL, 7.9G FIBRE AND 21.0G PROTEIN PER SERVING

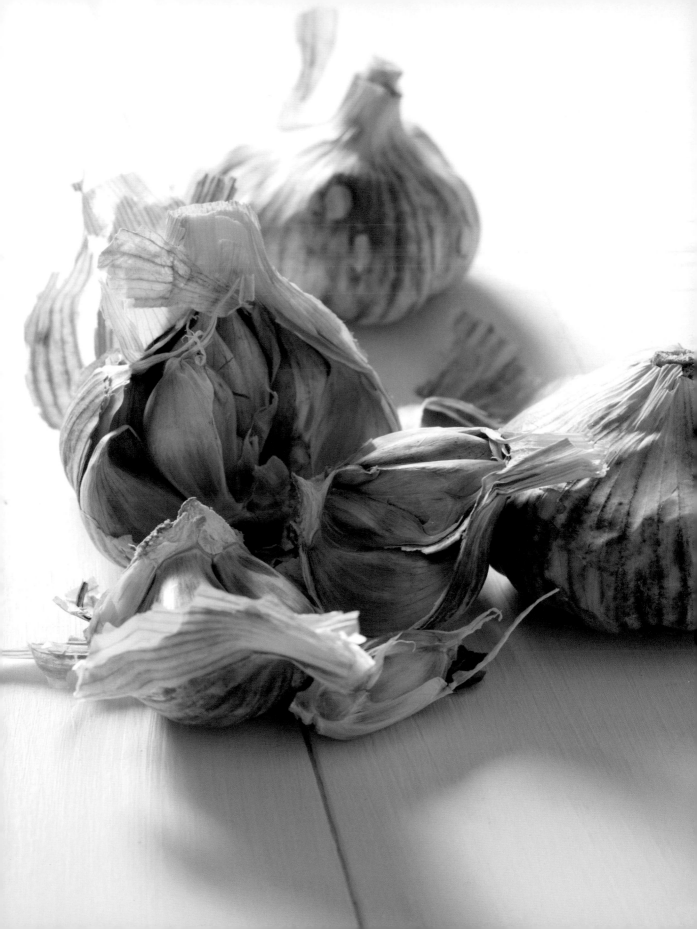

Snacks, Sides and Drinks

Over the years, I have met so many people who never actually eat a meal: they just snack all day long! This is obviously not good for your health – you must have regular meals every day to stay well.

Having said that, snacks play a small but important role in our diets: they fill the gap in between the meals, and in this way they help us to balance blood sugars.

So there is no problem with snacking – what matters is what you are snacking on! You need to have plenty of options: hot, cold, sweet and savoury. These recipes cover it all. Some are pâtés and spreads that are perfect when you want to liven up a meal. Some are baked treats that you can prepare ahead and stash away for whenever you need an energy boost. Some are dips, crudités and other nibbles that are lovely if friends call over for a visit. And there are lots of drinks too: hot or cold, with or without alcohol, depending on what you like. With all of these recipes, you will never be stuck for something to snack on.

Great Grandma's Berry Soup (Kiisseli)

The combination of rhubarb and strawberry works very well here. This berry soup also contains kuzu, a wonderful thickening agent that comes in powder form – it is a staple in my cupboard.

Have a snack like this ready in the fridge at all times – then you won't have to worry about sweet cravings. But this *kiisseli* is not just for you. Make this even for family and friends – I guarantee you they will love it! **Serves 4**

5 rhubarb stalks, finely chopped and covered with 1 litre of water
750g frozen strawberries
4 tbsp stevia (or more if you like it sweeter)
7 tbsp kuzu, diluted in 100ml cold water

Bring the rhubarb to the boil and cook, uncovered, for about 7 minutes. Stir in the frozen strawberries and stevia and return to the boil. Gradually pour in the kuzu, stirring to ensure the mixture is runny (not lumpy). Ladle the kiisseli into serving bowls and serve warm. Otherwise, place the bowls in the fridge until the kiisseli has cooled down.

APPROXIMATELY 147 KCAL, 16.1G FIBRE AND 3.9G PROTEIN PER SERVING

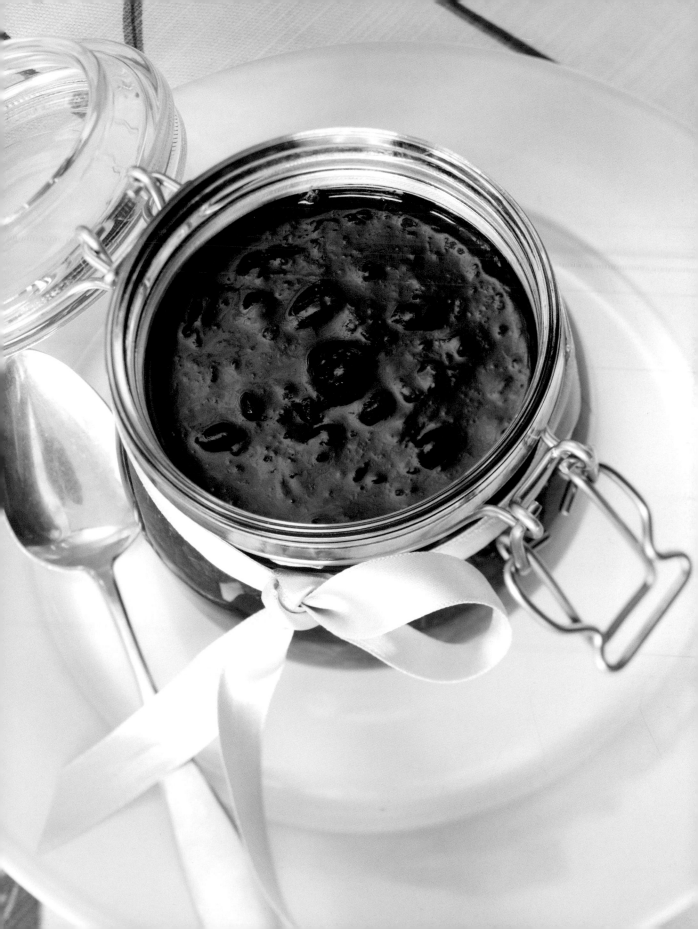

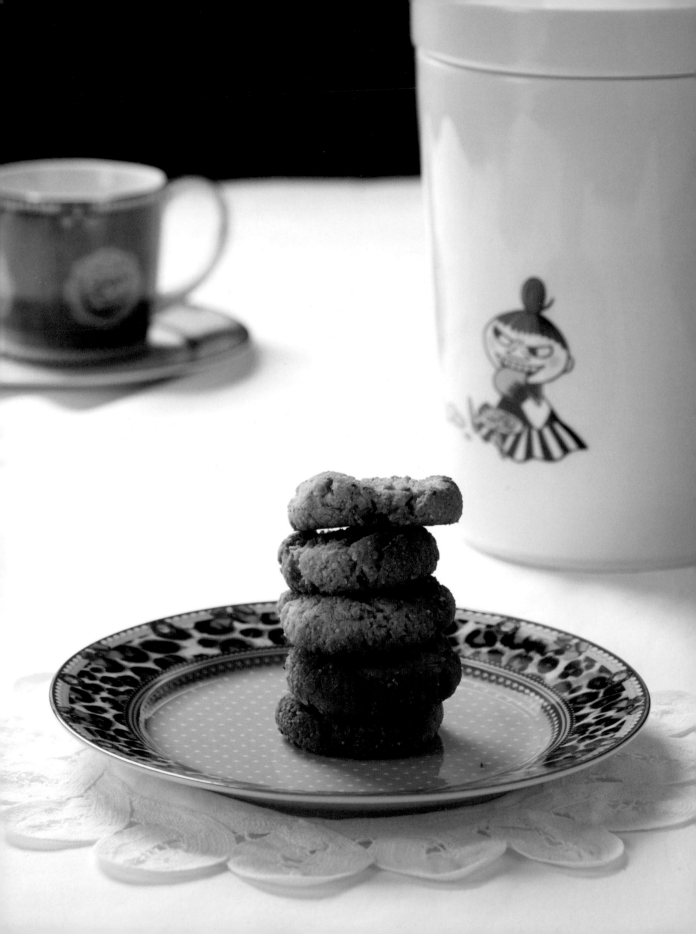

Coconut Biscuits

These biscuits have all the goodness of high-quality ingredients, unlike their cheap competitors in supermarkets! They are gluten-free and they keep well if stored in airtight containers. **Makes about 30 cookies**

200g buckwheat flakes
50g ground almonds
100g desiccated coconut
100g gram flour
1 tsp baking powder
A pinch of salt
½ tsp cinnamon
85g coconut oil
90ml maple syrup
75ml stevia
1 egg, lightly beaten
1 tsp vanilla extract

Preheat the oven to 160°C/325°F/gas 3. Line two large baking sheets with parchment paper.

Mix the buckwheat flakes, ground almonds, desiccated coconut, gram flour, baking powder, salt and cinnamon in a large bowl and set aside.

The coconut oil is solid at room temperature, so heat it in a small saucepan until the oil has just melted. Mix the melted coconut oil with the maple syrup and stevia in a large bowl. Add the egg and vanilla extract and mix until combined.

Pour the dry ingredients into the wet ingredients and mix well to form a firm cookie dough. Roll tablespoons of dough into a ball with your hands, then place them on the baking sheets and squish them down with a fork. Bake for 12 minutes and allow the cookies to cool slightly on the trays before removing to a wire rack.

APPROXIMATELY 126 KCAL, 1.1G FIBRE AND 1.6G PROTEIN PER SERVING (27G)

Carrot and Beetroot Muffins

Look – I am even able to get vegetables into muffins! You may not be familiar with all of the ingredients, but your local health food shop should stock them. These muffins should take care of your 'sweet tooth' cravings. **Makes 12 large muffins**

150g ground almonds
5 tbsp coconut flour
1 tsp cinnamon
1 tsp baking powder
8 tbsp coconut oil
4 eggs
80ml runny honey
2 tsp stevia
1 tsp vanilla extract
2 carrots, grated
4 beetroot, grated

Preheat the oven to 180°C/350°F/gas 4. Line a 12-bun muffin tin with muffin papers.

Combine the ground almonds, coconut flour, cinnamon and baking powder in a medium bowl and set aside.

The coconut oil is solid at room temperature, so heat it in a small pan until the oil has just melted. Meanwhile, whisk the eggs in a large bowl for a few minutes. Then stir in the honey, stevia, vanilla extract and melted coconut oil.

Pour the dry ingredients into the egg mixture and stir until just combined. Fold in the grated carrots and beetroot.

Spoon the mixture into the muffin papers and bake for 20–25 minutes, until the muffins are firm but moist. Carefully remove the muffins from the tin and allow to cool on a wire rack.

APPROXIMATELY 135 KCAL, 1.4G FIBRE and 4.3G PROTEIN PER SERVING

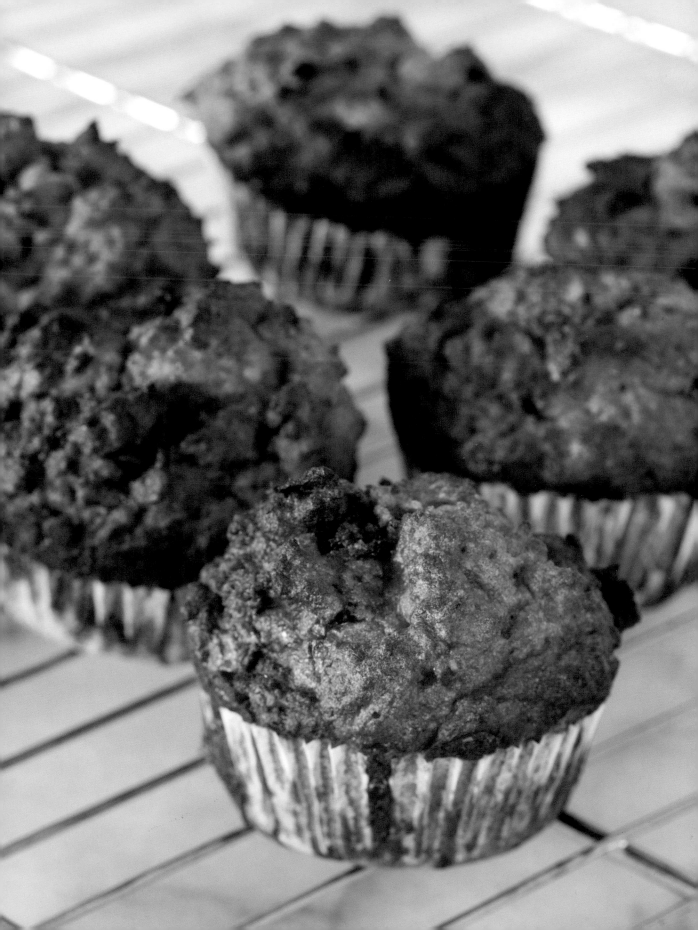

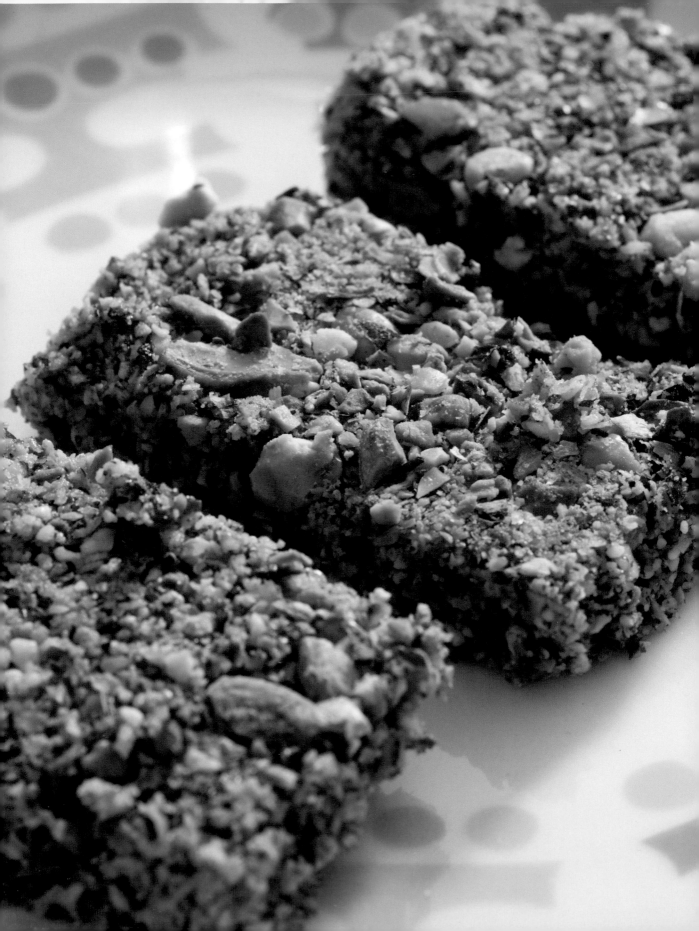

Granola Protein Bars

Everybody loves bars like these. They can be handy at breakfast time if you've slept in or are in a rush. Keep them wrapped up in the fridge to avoid temptation. And when you are in the middle of making them, don't pick at the ingredients!

It really makes a difference if you use toasted coconut flakes, so make the effort to go to your local health food shop to buy them and the other ingredients – you will be rewarded.
Makes 22 bars

100g coconut oil
50ml maple syrup
100g wheat-free oat bran
100g cashew nuts, chopped
100g brazil nuts, chopped
50g shelled pistachio nuts
50g flaxseeds
50g chia seeds
100g toasted coconut flakes
100g dried cranberries

Line a 33cm x 23cm (13 inch x 9 inch) metal baking tin with parchment paper.

Heat the coconut oil and maple syrup in a small pan over a low heat, stirring gently until combined. Remove from the heat and set aside.

Meanwhile, place the oat bran, cashew nuts, brazil nuts and pistachio nuts in a non-stick pan and toast over a low heat until golden. Remove the toasted nuts to the large heatproof bowl of an electric mixer. Pour in the flaxseeds, chia seeds, toasted coconut flakes and dried cranberries. Pour in the coconut and maple syrup and mix on a low setting with the paddle attachment for 30 seconds, or until just combined. Transfer to the prepared baking tin and spread out evenly, pressing down the mixture with the back of a spoon to make the surface as even as possible. Then cut the mixture into 22 bars, place the tin in the fridge and leave the bars to set overnight.

When the bars have set, wrap them individually in parchment paper or cling film – this makes portion control a lot easier! The bars keep for 7 days in the fridge and they also freeze well.

APPROXIMATELY 174 KCAL, 2.2G FIBRE AND 2.7G PROTEIN PER SERVING (36G)

Ultimate Health Loaf

Bread is not something I usually promote to people trying to lose weight. But weight reduction in the end is down to energy deficit. So, if you watch your portions, then yes – you can even have a slice of this delicious healthy rye-based bread. Just don't go over your calorie allowance for the day!

You need to make the dough and then leave it in a warm, draft-free place for 1 hour. At this point, I usually shout: 'Everybody keep the doors and windows closed – baby can't get cold!' When my family hears this, they know that something nice will be appearing on the table soon!

Serves 30 (Makes 3 loaves, each cut into 10 slices)

1 onion, roughly chopped
1 tbsp chopped fresh rosemary
1 tsp stevia
1 tsp salt
350ml light soya milk, warm
Olive oil
2 tsp (1 x 7g sachet) easy-blend (fast-action) yeast
300g organic rye flour
300g white spelt flour, plus extra for dusting the work surface
½ large butternut, peeled and cubed
200g feta, crumbled

Place the onion, rosemary and stevia in a large mixing bowl. Add the salt and 1 tablespoon of the warm soya milk and stir with a wooden spoon. Pour in the rest of the warm soya milk and mix well. Pour in 50ml olive oil and mix well. Mix the yeast with a little warm water, pour this in and mix well. Now add the flour, a few spoons at a time, mixing well after each addition. You can use the wooden spoon or your hands to mix in the flour. Gradually, it will come together to form a soft dough.

Flour the work surface and turn the dough out onto it. Knead the dough for a few minutes until it is smooth. Shape it into a neat ball, put it back in the mixing bowl and cover the bowl with a damp tea towel. Leave the bowl in a warm, draft-free place for 1 hour, until the dough has nearly doubled in size.

Meanwhile, preheat the oven to 180°C/350°F/gas 4. Rub three 18cm x 6cm (7 inch x 2.5 inch) loaf tins with a light coating of olive oil.

Use 1 teaspoon of olive oil to lightly coat the butternut cubes. Season and place them in a roasting tin. Roast for 15 minutes, until just tender. (Be careful not to overcook or the butternut will be mushy.) Remove from the oven and reduce the heat to 160°C/325°F/gas 3.

When the dough has risen, mix in the roasted butternut and feta. Lightly knead the dough, adding some extra flour, to create a longish rectangular shape. Then cut this into three so that the dough pieces fit nicely into the prepared tins. Bake for 60–70 minutes. Remember that this bread will be quite moist inside because of the feta and butternut. Remove from the oven and set aside to cool before serving.

APPROXIMATELY 60 KCAL, 2.6G FIBRE AND 3.6G PROTEIN PER SERVING

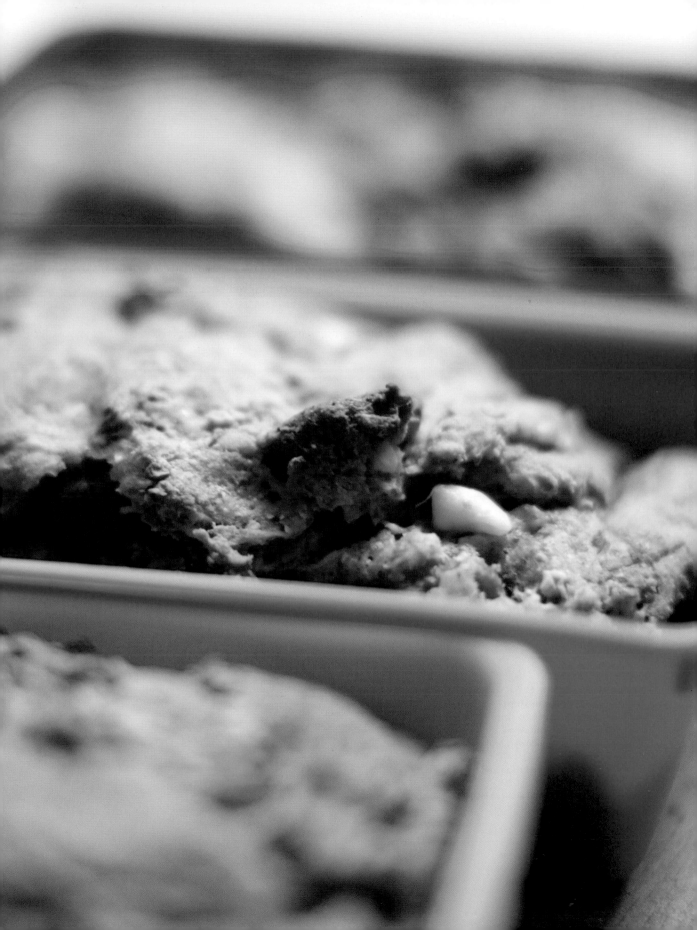

Crudités with Dips

When you have friends over, you might be tempted to tuck into crisps and cheeseboards – but don't! Make this crudités platter instead.

You can make three different dips with just one 500ml tub of natural yoghurt – make sure to find one with a very low calorie content. And you can use any raw vegetables you like. Choose a mixture of colours to get a range of antioxidants and flavours – and make sure to chew well! **Serves 4**

FOR THE TABASCO DIP
165g low fat natural yoghurt
2 tsp tomato ketchup
10 drops of Tabasco sauce
A pinch of salt
A pinch of black pepper

FOR THE HORSERADISH AND HERB DIP
165g low fat natural yoghurt
2 tsp mustard
2 tsp horseradish sauce
A pinch of salt
A pinch of black pepper
A handful of chopped fresh herbs (basil, parsley, thyme and coriander work well)

FOR THE CURRY DIP
165g low fat natural yoghurt
1 garlic clove, crushed
1 tsp medium curry powder
1 tsp soy sauce
½ tsp garam masala
½ tsp mustard
½ tsp stevia
A pinch of salt
A pinch of black pepper

FOR THE CRUDITÉS
4 carrots, cut into strips
4 celery sticks, cut into strips
1 large cucumber, cut into strips
1 large pepper, cut into strips
400g broccoli or cauliflower, broken into small florets
100g mushrooms, wiped clean and finely sliced
100g radishes, scrubbed and cut into strips

For each of the dips, mix the ingredients in an individual serving bowl and set aside.

Arrange the crudités and dips on a serving platter – and enjoy.

APPROXIMATELY 156 KCAL, 8.5G FIBRE AND 11.8G PROTEIN PER SERVING

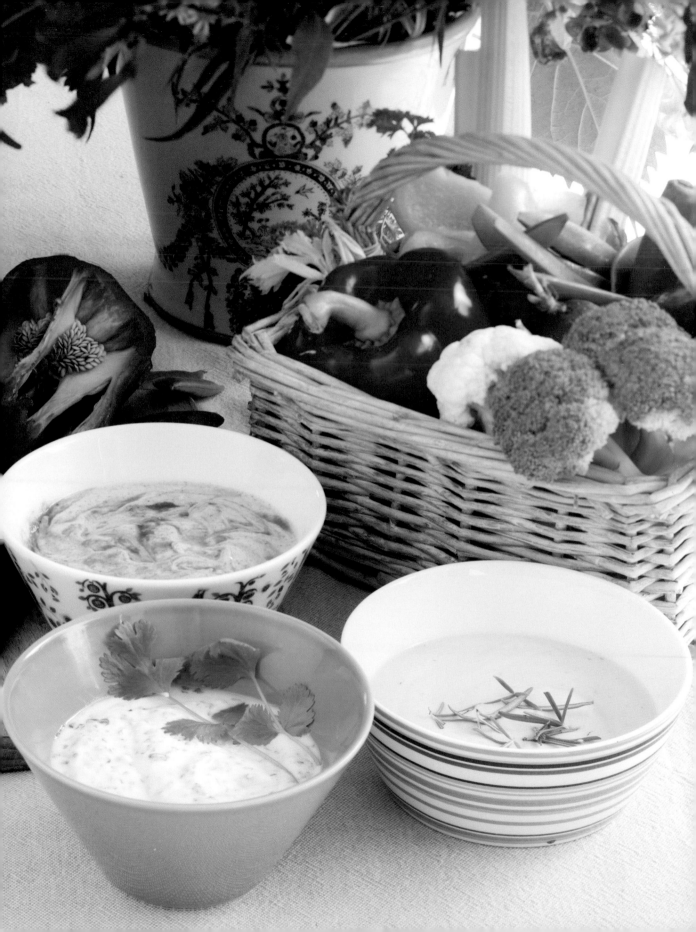

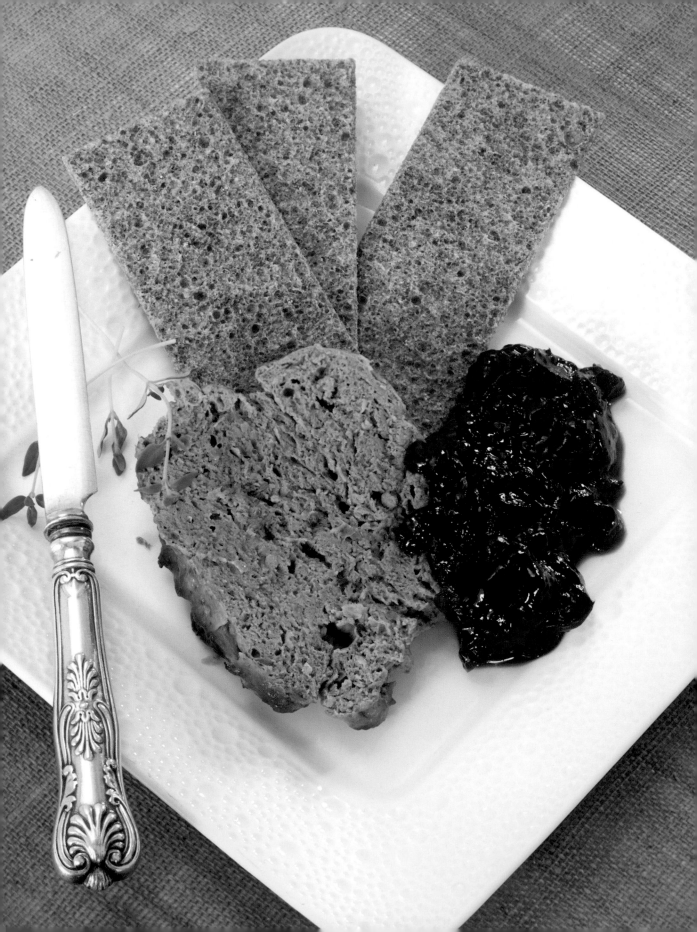

Finnish Pâté (Maksapasteija)

One of my favourite childhood foods was maksamakkara (liver pâté sausage) served on a slice of crusty French bread. Since I can't get that here in Ireland, I had to invent my own recipe for Finnish pâté (maksapasteija) to get my fix.

This recipe is easy to prepare once you have the right ingredients. It's best to prepare it in advance, so make it on a Sunday and then you have it for the busy week ahead.

You can serve it warm with a tablespoon of lingonberry jam and a green salad, the way we do in Finland. Or you could bulk it up with some steamed baby potatoes if you can spare the calories. **Serves 2**

250g minced pork
250g minced lamb
200g chicken livers, chopped
2 garlic cloves, chopped
1 onion, chopped
1 tbsp vegetable bouillon powder (or similar vegetable stock in powder form)
1 egg, lightly beaten
1 tbsp dried thyme
½ tbsp sugar
½ tsp salt
¼ tsp black pepper
10 green olives, stuffed with peppers (optional)

Preheat the oven to 160°C/325°F/gas 3. Grease a 900g (2lb) loaf tin or a 23cm x 13cm (9 inch x 5 inch) terrine dish.

Place all of the ingredients, except the olives, in a food processor and blend until smooth. If you can't fit everything in the food processor at once, do it in batches and then mix everything together in a large bowl.

Scrape the pâté mixture into the prepared tin. Push the olives into the mixture and cover the tin with foil. Place the tin in a large roasting tray half filled with water (this will keep the pâté moist in the oven). Bake for 1½–2 hours, until the pâté is firm. Leave to cool completely, then refrigerate.

APPROXIMATELY 278 KCAL, 1.0G FIBRE AND 35.4G PROTEIN PER SERVING

You can serve a slice (60g) of this pâté cold as a snack with three crispbreads (such as Finn Crisp) and a tablespoon of lingonberry jam. Cut the pâté into 12 portions (a 60g portion is approximately 103 KCAL).

The above snack (with the crispbreads) has approximately 195 KCAL, 5.2g fibre and 14.1g protein.

As an alternative, serve three slices of this pâté as a main meal with 150g steamed baby potatoes, one grated carrot and one tablespoon of lingonberry jam.

APPROXIMATELY 475 KCAL, 5.2G FIBRE AND 36G PROTEIN

Smoked Mackerel Pâté

This pâté goes really well with a freshly prepared crudité platter. It's also delicious with crispbreads. **Makes 20 tablespoons**

150g ricotta
90g smoked mackerel fillet, skin removed, chopped
⅓ cucumber, deseeded
2 tbsp soured cream
1 tbsp lemon juice
2 tsp horseradish sauce
A pinch of cayenne pepper

Place all of the ingredients in a food processor and blend until smooth.

APPROXIMATELY 30 KCAL, 0.1G FIBRE AND 1.6G PROTEIN PER SERVING (19G)

Creamy Salmon Pâté

This pâté is a perfect accompaniment to the Ultimate Health Loaf (p.174) and it is also great as a filler for a baked potato. I love having this pâté to serve when visitors call – it just feels elegant. **Makes 14 tablespoons**

150g boneless salmon, baked, cooled and flaked
100g low fat cream cheese
3 tsp capers
1 shallot, chopped
2 tbsp low fat crème fraîche
1 tbsp lemon juice
1 tbsp finely chopped fresh herbs (dill and parsley are good)
1–2 tsp mustard
A pinch of paprika
A pinch of salt

Place all of the ingredients in a food processor and blend until smooth.

APPROXIMATELY 39 KCAL AND 3.7G PROTEIN PER SERVING (23G)

Baba Ganoush

Baba ganoush can be used like hummus – on crisp bread or with crudités. There's really no work in this recipe: you bake the aubergine whole and then blitz everything in the food processor. So there really is no reason to be without a delicious low calorie spread. **Serves 4**

1 aubergine, whole
1 tbsp dark tahini paste
1 tbsp lemon juice
1 garlic clove, crushed
A pinch of salt
A pinch of chilli powder or paprika
A pinch of cumin
1 tbsp chopped flat-leaf parsley
    (optional)

Preheat the oven to 200°C/400°F/gas 6.

Place the aubergine on a baking tray and cook for 40–60 minutes, until tender. Remove from the oven and leave to cool down.

Cut the cooled aubergine in half lengthways and scrape out the flesh into a food processor. Add the rest of the ingredients and pulse until you have a smooth baba ganoush.

APPROXIMATELY 41 KCAL, 2.2G FIBRE AND 1.6G PROTEIN PER SERVING

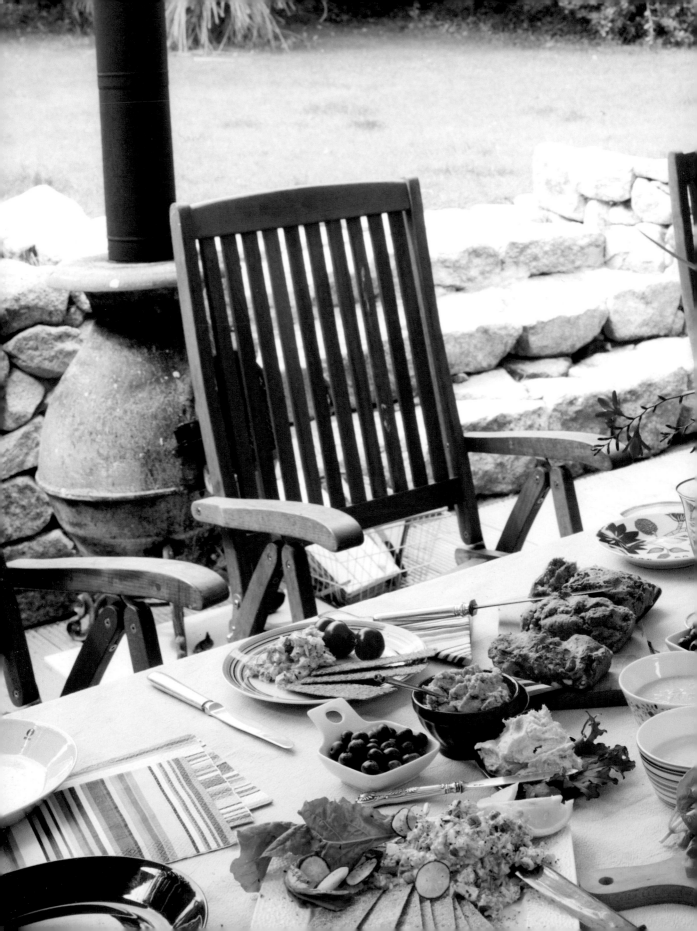

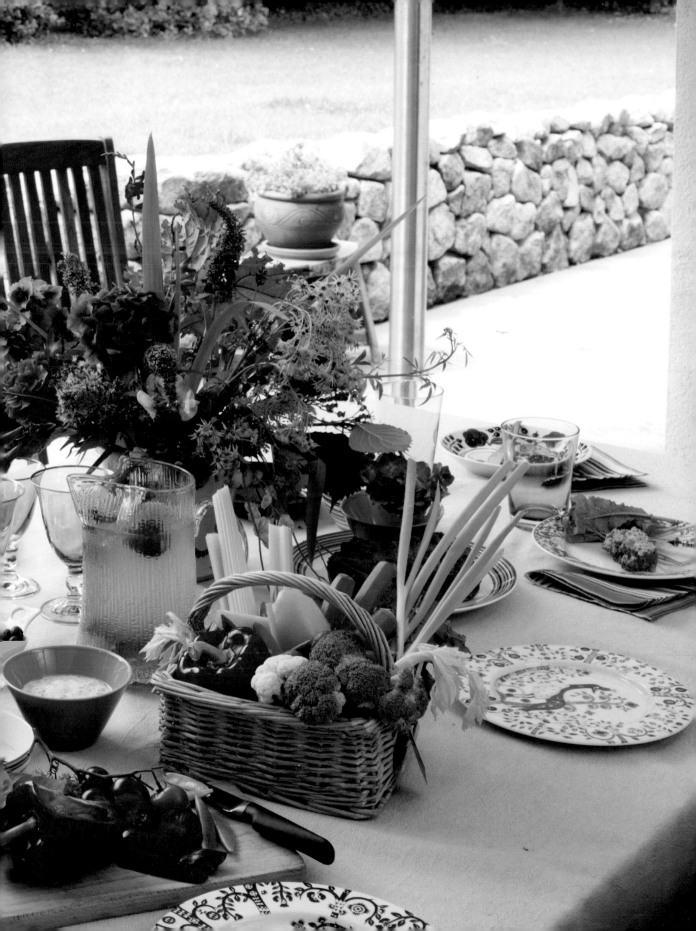

Cauliflower Mash

Who wouldn't like a substitute for mashed potatoes? I can honestly say that this mash goes just as well, if not better, alongside a steak or piece of roasted meat. If you want to make things really easy, use frozen cauliflower. **Serves 2**

1 cauliflower, broken into florets
75ml milk substitute (Laktolight) or light coconut milk
1 scallion, finely chopped
1 tbsp low fat cream cheese
1 tsp dried parsley
1 tsp garlic powder
1 tsp wholegrain mustard
Salt and freshly ground black pepper

Cook the cauliflower in a steamer until tender. Drain and place in a large bowl along with the milk substitute. Mash well and stir in the rest of the ingredients. Season to taste and serve.

APPROXIMATELY 160 KCAL, 8.8G FIBRE AND 13.9G PROTEIN PER SERVING

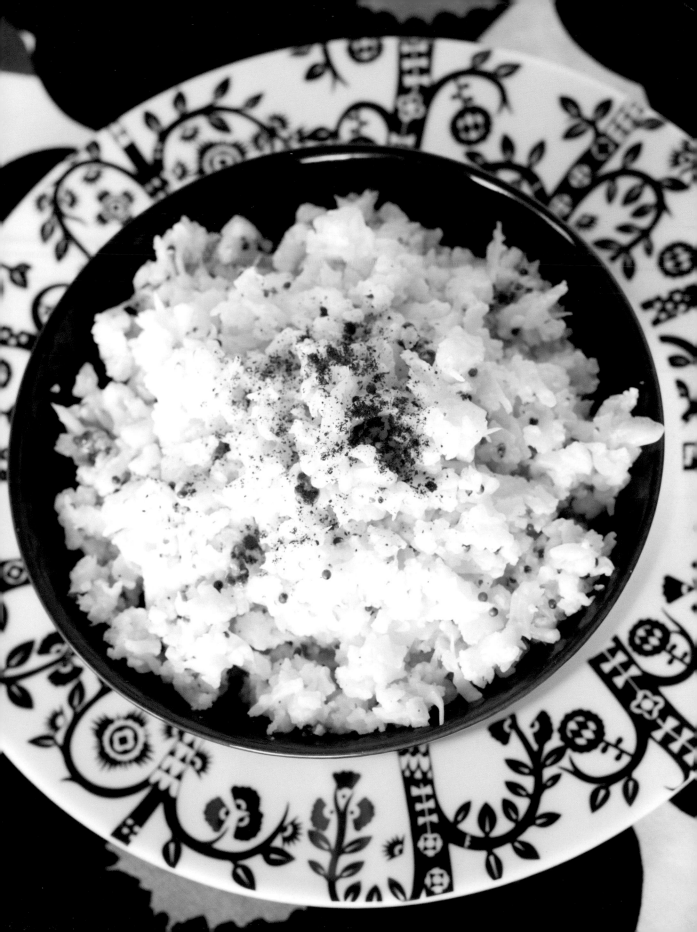

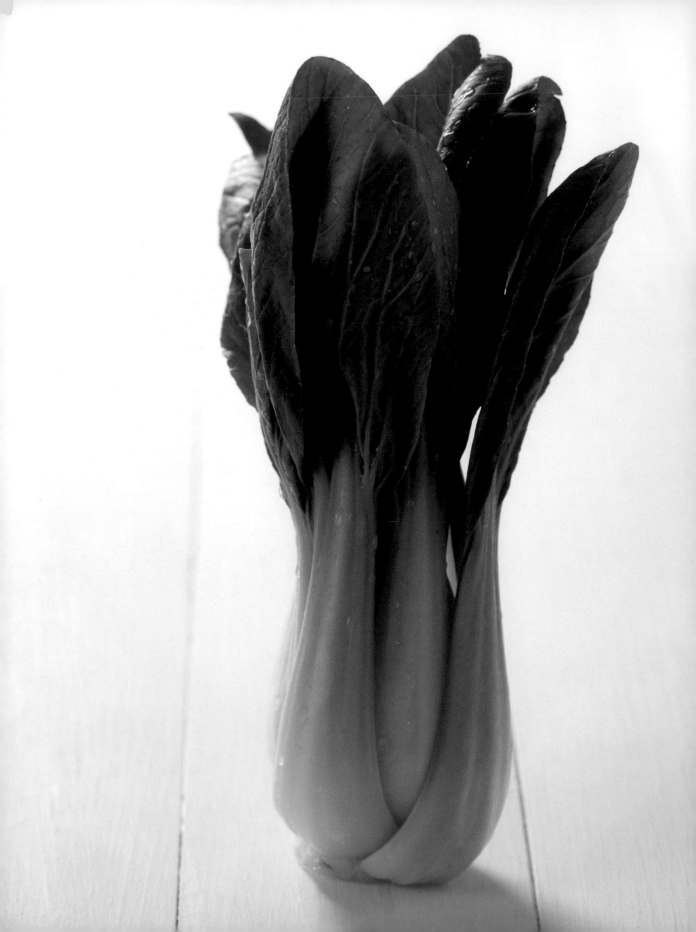

Pak Choi Stir-Fry

Choose smaller pak choi for better taste. It cooks very quickly, so add it in at the end when making stir-fries. You could also try it raw in salads – it provides real crunch. **Serves 4**

1 tbsp coconut oil
1 leek, finely sliced
1 tsp chilli paste
1 tsp ginger paste
100ml beef stock (you won't use all of this)
1 red pepper, finely sliced
1 green pepper, finely sliced
2–3 celery sticks, finely sliced
250g chestnut mushrooms, finely sliced
1 tbsp Worcestershire sauce
600g pak choi leaves, separated
160ml coconut milk (preferably organic)

Heat the coconut oil in a large pan over a medium heat. Add the leek, chilli paste and ginger paste and cook for 1 minute, stirring all the time. Add 1 tablespoon of stock, if the paste starts to catch. Add the peppers and celery and stir-fry for about 3 minutes, adding more stock if the vegetables start to catch. Add the mushrooms and Worcestershire sauce and stir-fry for 3–5 minutes, adding more stock if necessary. Add the pak choi and stir in the coconut milk. Leave to simmer for 2 minutes, then serve in warmed serving bowls.

APPROXIMATELY 173 KCAL, 2.9G FIBRE AND 5.1G PROTEIN PER SERVING

Courgette Hummus

It is a good idea to prepare this Courgette Hummus at the same time as the Baba Ganoush on p.181, since the vegetables need the same cooking time and there are similar ingredients in each recipe. The hummus is lovely spread on bread or used as a dip. **Serves 4**

1 large courgette, whole
1 garlic clove, crushed
1 tbsp dark tahini paste
1 tbsp lemon juice
4 tsp paprika
¼ tsp cumin
¼ tsp salt

Preheat the oven to 200°C/400°F/gas 6.

Place the courgette on a baking tray and cook for 40–60 minutes, until tender. Remove from the oven and leave to cool down.

Discard any charred flesh, then roughly chop the courgette and place it in a food processor. Add the rest of the ingredients and pulse until you have a smooth hummus.

APPROXIMATELY 50KCAL, 1.6G FIBRE AND 2.5G PROTEIN PER SERVING

High Fibre Salad

I'm always trying to remind my patients that salads on a weightloss journey can't be made up of lettuce, cucumber and tomato only: you need to add high fibre ingredients to increase bulk and prolong the feeling of fullness.

The combination of the colours in this salad makes it very aesthetically pleasing. Better still – if you use really fresh ingredients, this salad is good for several days.
Serves 4

300g white cabbage, finely sliced
300g red cabbage, finely sliced
8 cherry tomatoes, whole
½ large cucumber, deseeded and sliced
1 celery stick, sliced
½ red pepper, sliced
A handful of rocket

Mix all of the ingredients in a large salad bowl. Serve it with the Mustard and Anchovy Dressing on p.192 or another low calorie dressing of your choice.

APPROXIMATELY 58 KCAL, 4.7G FIBRE AND 2.9G PROTEIN PER SERVING

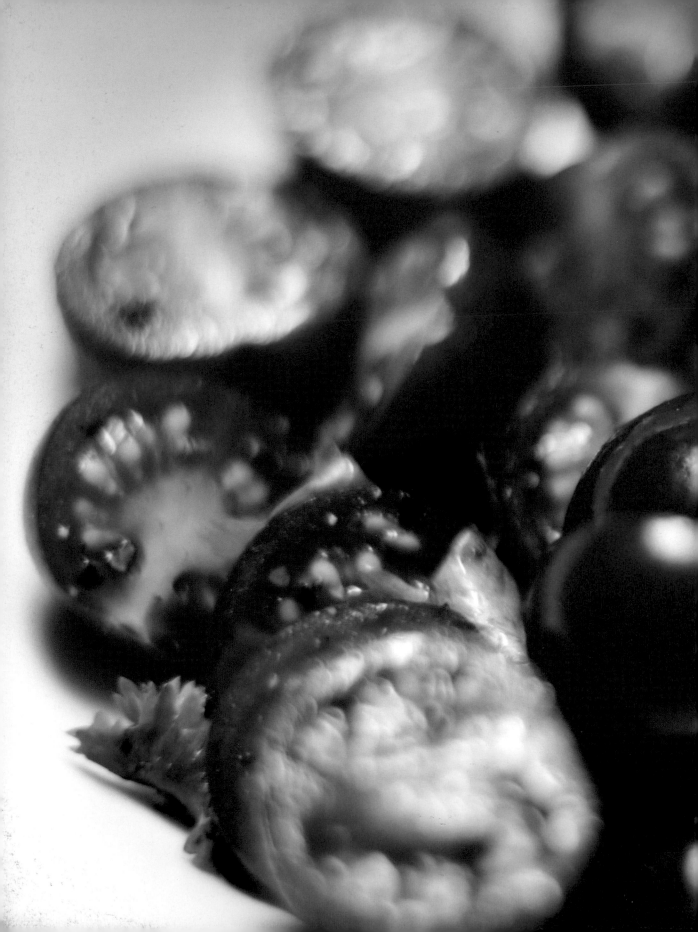

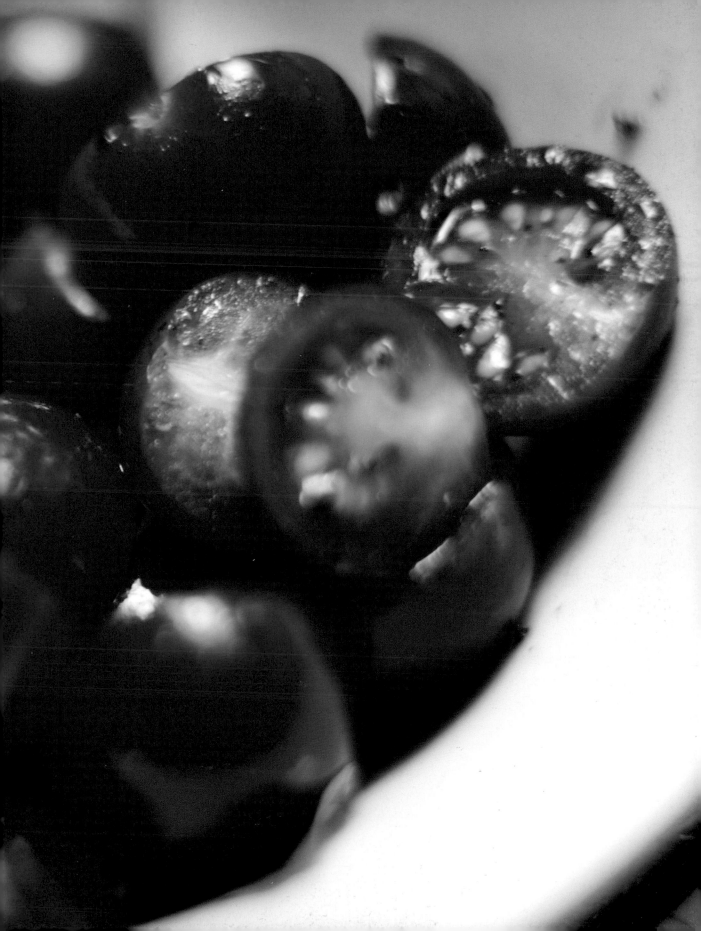

Mustard and Anchovy Dressing

This dressing is full of flavour – it can really bring life to all sorts of salads!
Serves 7

50ml rapeseed oil
50ml olive oil
50ml cider vinegar
2 egg yolks (room temperature)
1 tsp mustard
6 anchovies, drained and finely chopped

Mix the rapeseed oil and olive oil in a small jug and set aside.

Lightly whisk the cider vinegar, egg yolks and mustard in a medium bowl. Gradually pour in the oils, whisking continuously to blend. Add the anchovies, give everything a stir and serve.

APPROXIMATELY 138 KCAL AND 1.4G PROTEIN PER SERVING (31G)

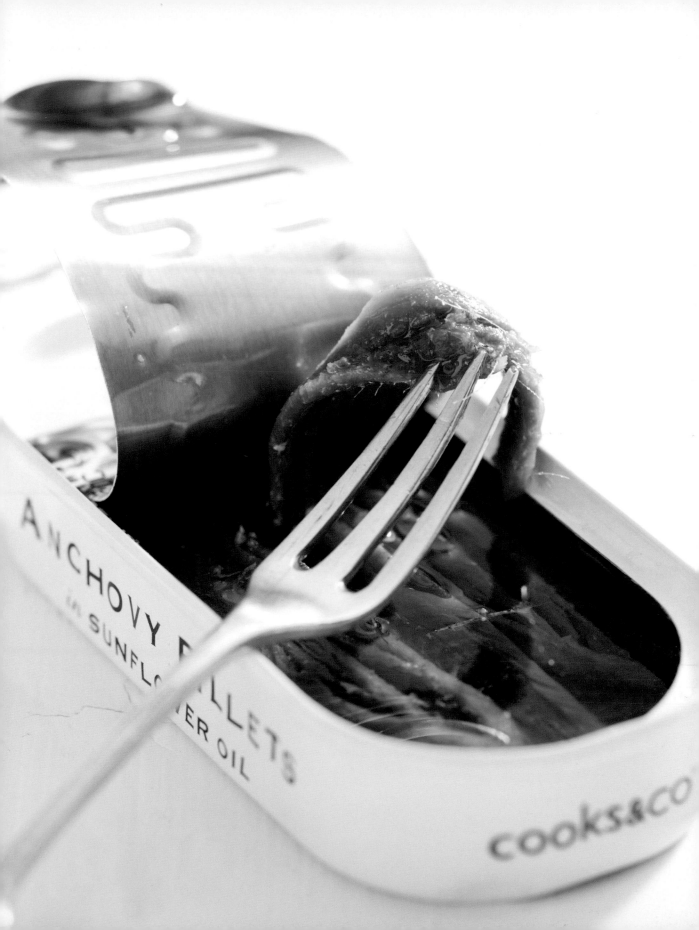

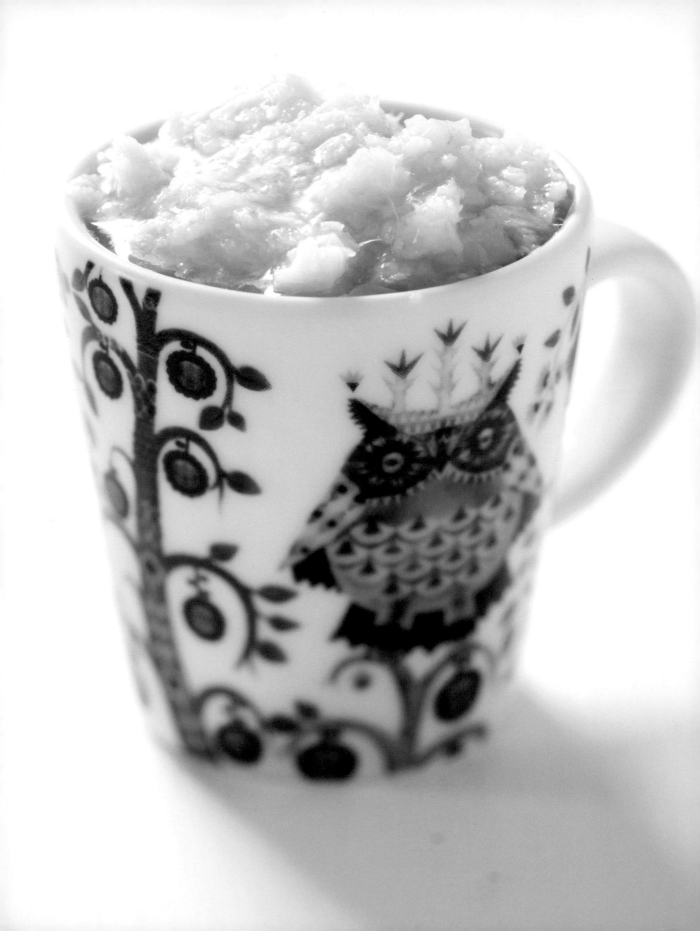

Ginger Garlic Paste

I use this paste all the time in my cooking. I first got the recipe from a patient – a lovely lady from Pakistan. It is such a clever idea to have ginger and garlic prepared in a paste like this. Whenever you want to make a stir-fry, it's ready to go!

Makes 20 tablespoons

100g garlic cloves, peeled and chopped
100g ginger, peeled and chopped
Olive oil

Place the garlic, ginger and 100ml olive oil in a food processor and blend until smooth. Scrape the paste into a sterilised glass jar, top with 50ml olive oil and close the lid. The paste will keep for weeks in the fridge.

APPROXIMATELY 65 KCAL, 0.1G FIBRE AND 0.5G PROTEIN PER SERVING (16G)

Mustard

Make a batch of this and use it in any of the recipes that call for some mustard – it's especially good in the Cauliflower Mash on p.184 but it also gives a lovely sweetness to salad dressings. The brandy also gives it a nice kick. **(Makes 7 tablespoons)**

1 egg, lightly beaten
3 tbsp low fat crème fraîche
2 tbsp stevia
2 tbsp mustard powder
½ tsp cornflour
1 tsp cider vinegar
1 tbsp brandy

Place the egg, crème fraîche, stevia, mustard powder and cornflour in a large pan over a medium heat. Whisk vigorously while the mixture heats up and becomes a smooth sauce. Remove from the heat and allow to cool down completely. Stir in the cider vinegar and brandy. Your mustard is ready to be bottled!

APPROXIMATELY 8 KCAL AND 2.5G PROTEIN PER SERVING (1 TSP)

Mayonnaise

My patients often think that mayonnaise is banned if they are on a diet. This is not true! My recipe for mayonnaise is a healthy alternative. I use rapeseed oil, which is a good source of omega-3 fatty acids. **(Makes 400ml)**

2 egg yolks
1 tbsp cider vinegar (preferably organic)
½ tsp salt
1 tsp mustard
50ml lukewarm water
200ml rapeseed oil

Blend all the ingredients except the oil in a food processor for about 15 seconds, or until well combined. While the motor is running, pour the oil into the food processor very slowly until the mayonnaise is well combined. Scrape the mayonnaise into a sterilised glass jar and close the lid. The mayonnaise will keep for a few weeks in the fridge.

APPROXIMATELY 65 KCAL AND 0.3G PROTEIN PER SERVING (1 TBSP)

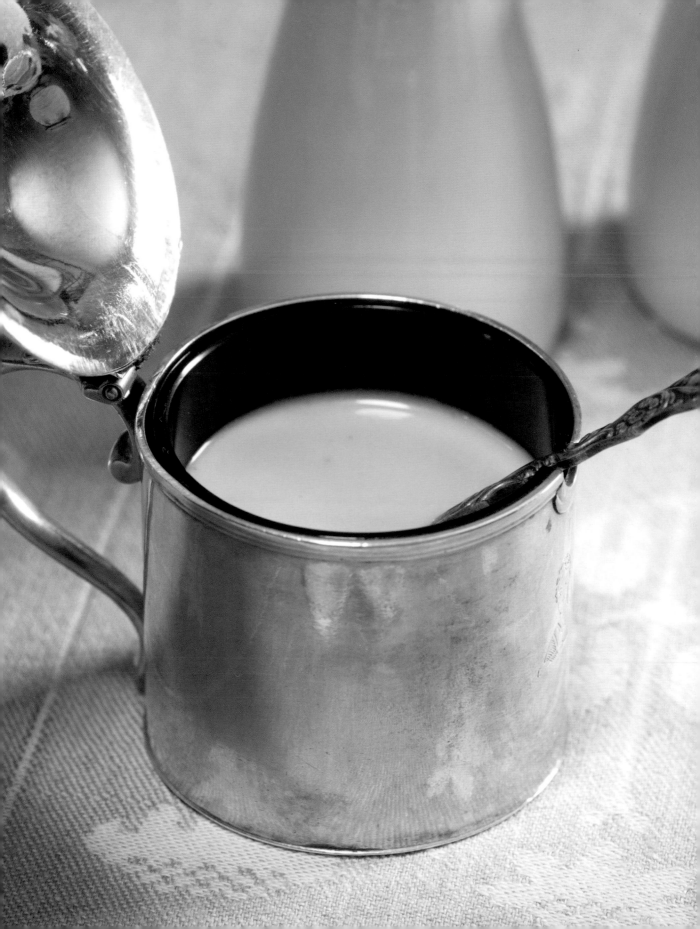

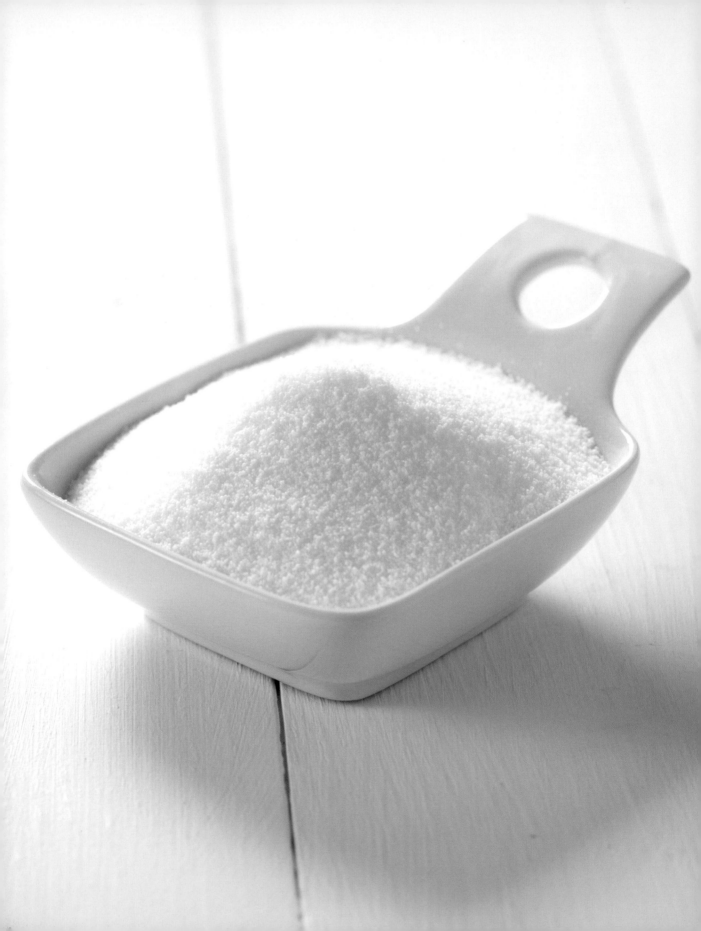

Earl Grey Iced Tea with Mint

This is really refreshing – especially on a warm day. The fresh mint and lemon provide a real zing! **Serves 8**

7cm piece of ginger, peeled and finely sliced
1 tbsp chopped fresh mint
1 tbsp Earl Grey tea, loose
1 tbsp stevia
1 litre boiling water
20–30 ice cubes
2 x 330ml cans of Diet 7 Up or soda water
Mint sprigs, to garnish
Lemon slices, to garnish

Place the ginger, mint, tea and stevia in a large teapot and pour in the boiling water. Leave to infuse for 15 minutes.

Meanwhile, divide the ice cubes between two jugs of 1¼ litre capacity. Pour the tea through a sieve, dividing it evenly between the two jugs. Pour a can of Diet 7 Up into each jug and stir. Garnish with fresh mint and lemon slices.

APPROXIMATELY 10 KCAL, 0.2G FIBRE AND 0.3G PROTEIN PER SERVING

Rooibos and Apple Iced Tea

Rooibos tea is known for its health benefits and this recipe adds extra flavour with apple and lemon. You can make a big batch of this and keep it in the fridge – it's a nice way to stay hydrated. **Serves 4**

2 rooibos tea bags
1 cooking apple, peeled and finely
  chopped
2 litres boiling water
2–4 tsp stevia
Juice of 2 lemons
Grated rind of 2 lemons (optional)

Place the tea bags and apple in a large teapot and pour in the boiling water. Sprinkle in the stevia and leave for 10 minutes so that the tea infuses and cools down.

Stir in the lemon juice and rind and serve warm – or leave to stand for several minutes and serve cool.

APPROXIMATELY 16 KCAL, 0.8G FIBRE AND 0.1G PROTEIN PER SERVING

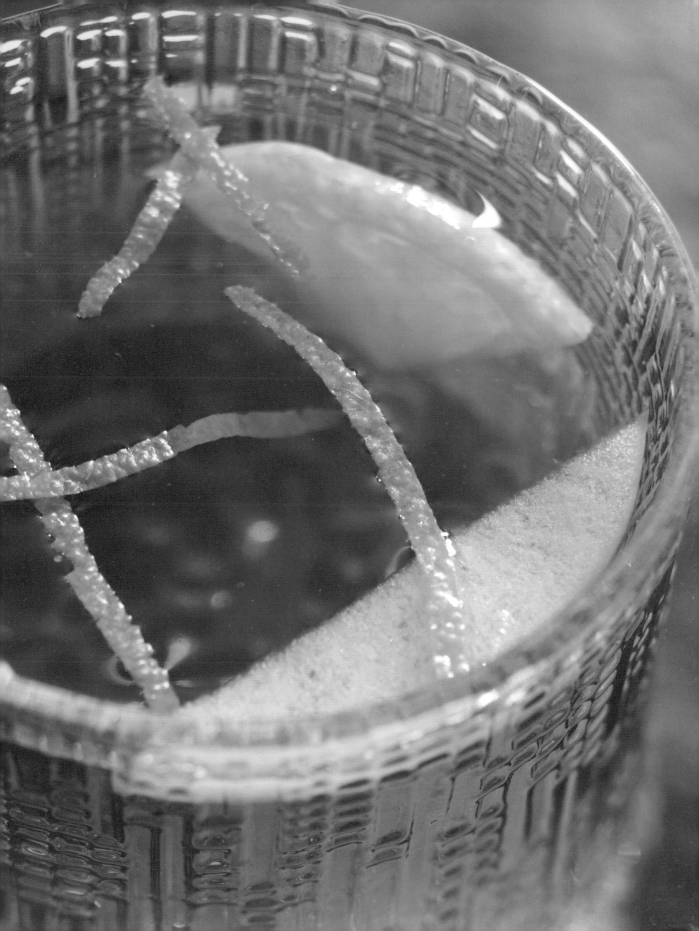

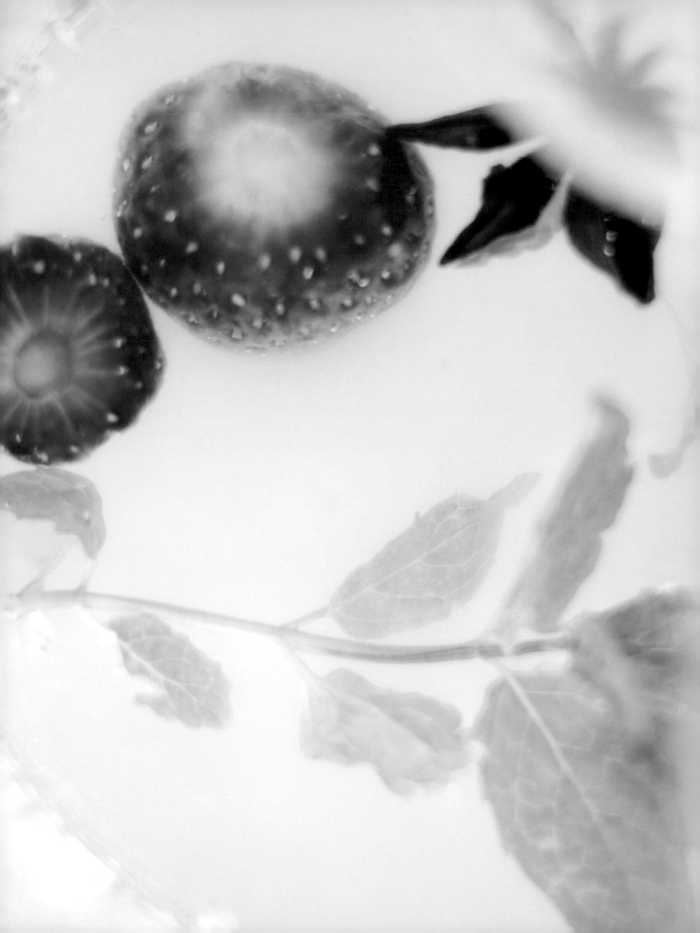

White Wine Sangria

This sangria will allow you to enjoy some white wine without going over the top with calories or alcohol. Adding the ice and other ingredients means that you 'stretch out' the wine and the rum so that you can enjoy them guilt-free. Feel free to garnish this with star anise, mint or even strawberries! **Serves 8**

1 litre white wine
500ml freshly squeezed orange juice
300ml rum
3 apples, finely sliced
1 lemon, finely sliced
2 tbsp stevia
Ice cubes, to serve

Mix all of the ingredients in a large jug and add plenty of ice, to serve.

APPROXIMATELY 221 KCAL, 1.3G FIBRE AND 0.7G PROTEIN PER SERVING

Hot Chocolate

Even when we are on a diet, we sometimes need a chocolate fix. This hot chocolate drink is a smart way to indulge! **Serves 1**

200ml dairy-free coconut milk, such as
   Koko
1 tsp Bourneville cocoa powder
Stevia
Vanilla extract

Warm the milk and blend in the cocoa powder. Add stevia and vanilla extract to taste.

APPROXIMATELY 84 KCAL, 1.7G FIBRE AND 1.2G PROTEIN PER SERVING

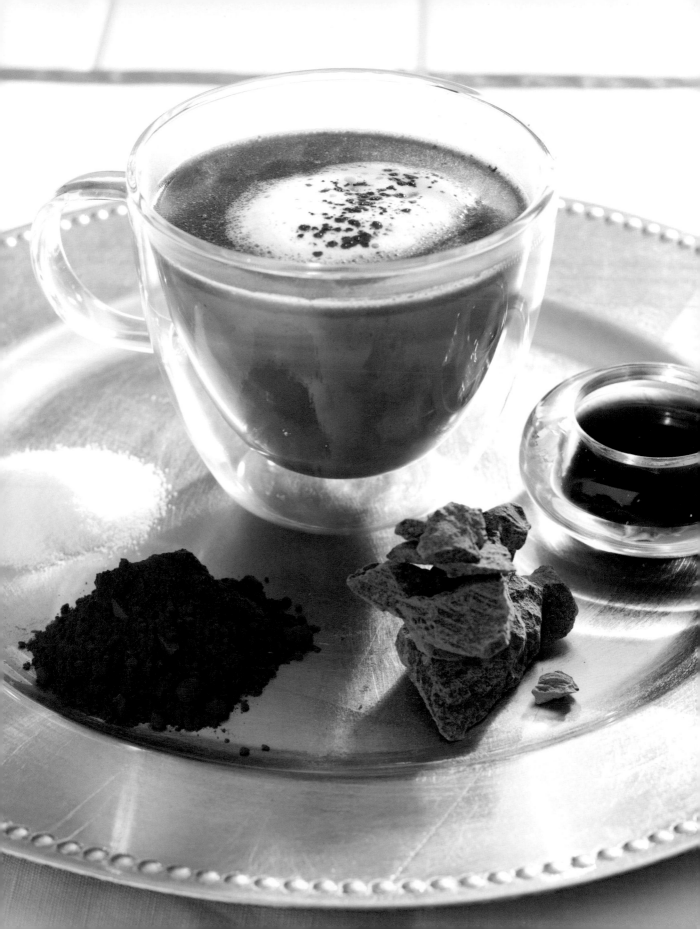

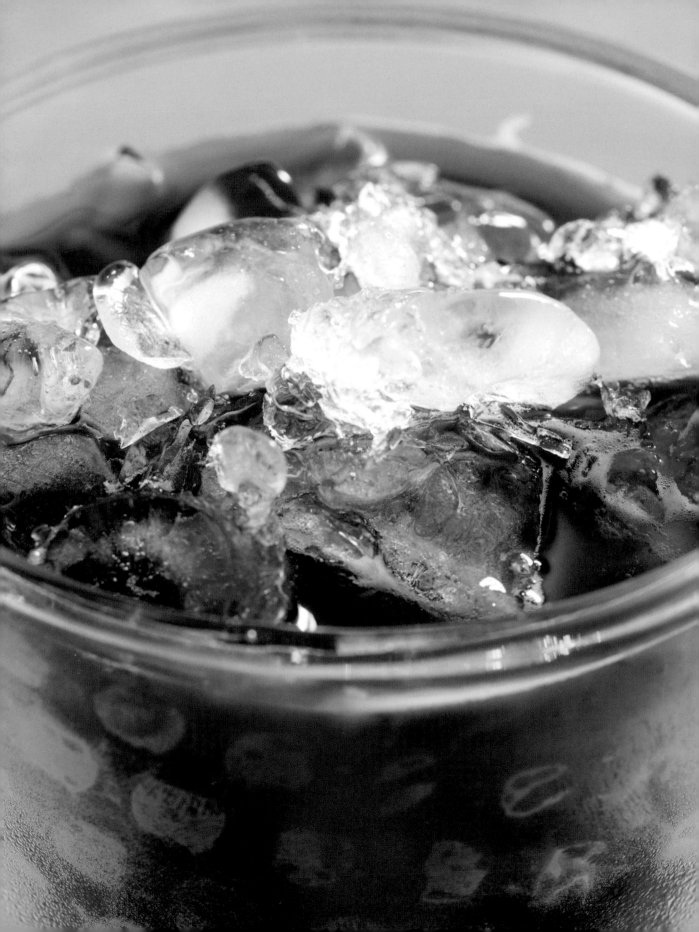

Italian-Style Coffee

Moderate coffee intake (2–3 cups a day) can be beneficial to your health, since coffee is a powerful antioxidant. Some research indicates that coffee drinkers are less likely to get Type 2 diabetes than non-coffee drinkers. The jury is still out – but you can't go wrong if you enjoy things in moderation.

Scandinavians are serious coffee drinkers. As well as being a Finn, I lived in Italy for seven years, so coffee is certainly part of my day. I need my fix especially in the morning so that I can get going!

I invested in an Italian coffee machine that grinds the fresh coffee beans and makes my espresso, but you can use strongly-brewed coffee for any of the recipe ideas below. I also have a special milk frother that makes beautiful thick foam – I highly recommend you buy one of those! You can experiment in many different ways to create Italian-Style Coffee. **Serves 1**

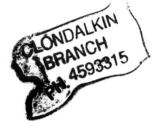

My morning fix is a **Light Soya Cappuccino** made with one espresso and 100ml light soya milk. It has just 22 kcal and you don't need to add any sweetener, since the light soya milk is already sweet!

If I feel like having a latte, I make a **Light Soya Latte** with one espresso and 200ml light soya milk. It comes to just 44 kcal.

And I make **Iced Coffee** when I entertain or when I want to cheat myself into thinking that something with virtually no calories is in reality an amazing treat! I use a cocktail shaker to mix one espresso with lots of crushed ice. You could add a teaspoon of stevia, if you need to. Whatever you do, use an elegant glass (even a Martini glass!) so that it feels like a real treat.

UNUSUAL INGREDIENTS

Regular shops and supermarkets should be able to provide you with most of the ingredients for my recipes. However, it is a good idea to visit local health food shops and Asian food stores to stock up on any of the more unusual ingredients. Look out for the following ingredients and stock up on them whenever you can!

COCONUT OIL

Coconut oil has been consumed in tropical countries for thousands of years. It is sold in glass jars and it is usually solid at room temperature (except on hot days!) since it has a melting point of 24°C. A lot of health claims have been made for its properties – from anti-viral to anti-cancer – but I love it for its sweet flavour and for the smell in the kitchen when I use it for stir-fries or baking.

DAIRY-FREE COCONUT MILK (KOKO)

This milk is naturally free from lactose and gluten. It is pressed from coconuts and is substantially lower in calories (27 kcal per 100ml) than semi-skimmed milk (47 kcal per 100ml). Please don't confuse dairy-free coconut milk with the coconut milk (typically sold in cans) that is used to flavour stir-fries and curries – that has a much higher calorie and fat content!

FLOUR SUBSTITUTES

Coconut flour is gluten-free, low in carbohydrates and high in fibre. These characteristics, along with its lovely flavour, make coconut flour an ideal ingredient for baking. Try my Carrot and Beetroot Muffins (p.170) and you will know what I mean! Spelt flour is an ancient grain. It is wonderfully nutritious and it has a deep nutty flavour – but remember that it does contain gluten. Gram flour is made from ground chickpeas and is naturally gluten-free.

HERBAMARE HERBAL SALT

This is a blend of sea salt with different herbs and vegetables, and it is MSG-free. When I want a quick snack, I sprinkle it over cucumber and tomato slices on thin crisp breads such as Finn Crisp. Herbamare always enhances the flavour of dishes, which means you end up using less salt.

KONNYAKU NOODLES

These noodles are made from the root of the Konjac yam. Konnyaku noodles (sometimes called shirataki noodles) are thin, translucent, gelatinous Asian noodles. They are very low in calories and are claimed to have no starch, no sugar and no protein.

KUZU

This is a high-quality organic starch that is extracted from the roots of a Japanese wild plant. In Japan and China, kuzu is well known for its medicinal properties. It can be used to thicken soups, stews and sauces.

MRS H.S. BALL'S CHUTNEY

I discovered Mrs H.S. Ball's Chutney during my South African years. It is one of my husband's favourites, and so I have started adding it to stews and stir-fries for extra flavour!

OILS

I believe it is worth spending money on good olive oil, which is readily available nowadays. Rapeseed oil is a great substitute for olive oil, and now we have Irish rapeseed oil as well. Buy a spray container and fill it with your favourite oil: this will help to control the quantity and the calories.

POMEGRANATE MOLASSES

This is a concentrated form of pomegranate juice, so a little goes a long way! It is tangy and sweet and is an essential ingredient in traditional Middle Eastern cooking.

STEVIA

This plant-based sugar substitute is unlike artificial sweeteners (e.g. aspartame). It has no significant calorific value and it can be used to sweeten many dishes. Porridge is delicious with the addition of ½ teaspoon of stevia and 1 teaspoon of cinnamon or cocoa powder. Stevia can also be used with soy sauce to give stir-fries and curries a delicious kick! It has been used in South America for centuries.

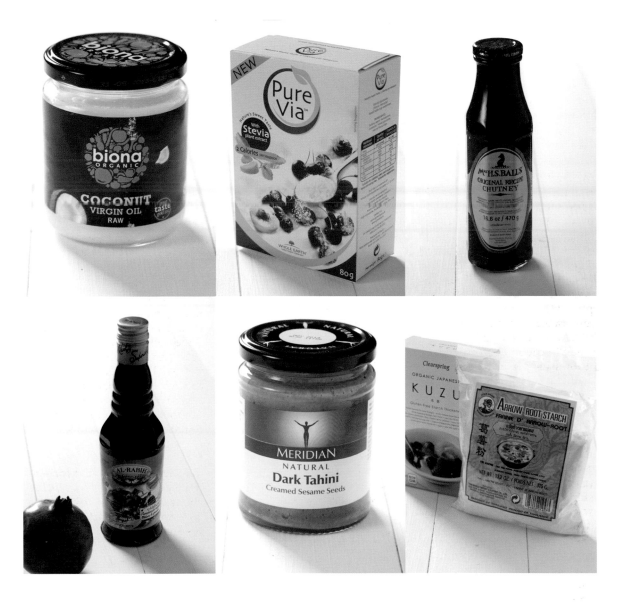

SUMAC
This tangy, crimson spice is commonly used in Middle Eastern cuisine to add a lemony taste to salads and meats. It is also widely used as a garnish on meze dishes in Arab, Turkish and Persian cuisine. Sumac is the spice that gives the special flavour to my Turkish Pizza (p.114).

TAHINI PASTE
This is a sesame seed paste with a nutty flavour. It is used in my Baba Ganoush (p.181) and Courgette Hummus (p.188). It is rich in protein and healthy fats, and has only a trace of sugar. The taste is strong – so you only need a small amount!

WASABI
Wasabi and horseradish are similar – but wasabi is green and is hotter in flavour. Because the base plant is difficult to cultivate, wasabi is expensive. Its root is used as a condiment and it has a very strong taste. Wasabi is sold in powder form or in tubes of ready-to-use paste.

INDEX

alcohol 6, 15

baba ganoush 181
bacon and halloumi stew 117
baked beans 106
baked trout 129
banana pancake 40
barley porridge (ohraryynipuuro) 37
beef, pomegranate and, casserole 108
berry soup, Great Grandma's 166
biscuits, coconut 169
Bolognese, chilli 158
borscht 81
bread 174
breakfast, generally 33
buckwheat flatbreads 45
burgers, turkey, with celeriac chips 130

cabbage soup, Mima's 66
calorie requirements 9
cappuccino, light soya 207
carbonara, cauliflower, easy 161
carrot and beetroot muffins 170
casserole, pomegranate and beef 108
cauliflower
  carbonara, easy 161
  mash 184
  scrambled eggs 44
celeriac
  chips 130
  mushroom soup 71
celery Roquefort soup 76
chicken
  butternut bake 142
  fried rice 134
  kebabs, with pomegranate molasses 139
  soup, Chinese 90
  tacos, spicy 133
  tikka masala 140

chilli
  dipping sauce 60
  pasta Bolognese 158
Chinese chicken soup 90
chips, celeriac 130
chocolate, hot 204
chorizo soup, creamy 83
chutney, Mrs H. S. Ball's 112, 209
cigarettes 6
coconut
  biscuits 169
  milk 46, 209
  oil 209
coffee 207
  iced, Italian 207
courgette
  and bacon pancake 41
  bake 154
  hummus 188
cowboy stew 106
creamy chorizo soup 83
creamy ham and garlic pasta 162
creamy prawn risotto 125
creamy salmon pâté 180
crudités with dips 176
curry
  dip 176
  green, vegetable 152

dal, yellow 149
diabetes 7
Diet Diaries 22–9
dill-cured salmon tartare 58
dinner, generally 105
dips/dipping sauces
  chilli 60
  curry 176
  horseradish and herb 176
  peanut 60
  Tabasco 176
Dr Eva's eggs Benedict 34

Earl Grey iced tea with mint 199
easy cauliflower carbonara 161
easy fish pie 124

eggs
  Benedict, Dr Eva's 34
  scrambled: cauliflower 44; with caviar 48
energy levels, low 7
exercise(s) 16–21

fajitas, vegetable 150
farmer's pie 116
fast plan 10, 12–13, 24–6
Filler Soups 13, 57, 64–79
Finnish pâté (maksapasteija) 179
fish see also salmon, squid, sushi, trout
  with mushroom sauce 128
  pie, easy 124
  rolls 121
  soup 88
flatbreads, buckwheat 45
flaxseed 46
flours 209
fried halloumi and cumin-spiced leeks 145
fried rice, chicken 134

ginger garlic paste 195
glucose levels 7
granola protein bars 173
Great Grandma's berry soup 166
green curry, vegetable 152
guacamole 133

halloumi
  bacon and, stew 117
  fried, and cumin-spiced leeks 145
  salad, warm 96
ham and garlic pasta, creamy 162
health loaf, ultimate 174
Herbamare herbal salt 209
horseradish and herb dip 176
hot chocolate 204
hummus, courgette 188

iced coffee, Italian 207
iced tea
  Earl Grey, with mint 199
  rooibos and apple 200
insulin 7

juice, purple 'pick me up' 52

kebabs, chicken, with
  pomegranate molasses 139
Kegel exercises 20
kiisseli 37, 166
Konnyaku noodles 209
kuzu 209

lamb rogan josh 111
lasagne, 'now to wow' 157
leek and potato soup 91
lentils 149
light soya cappuccino 207
lunch, generally 57

mackerel, smoked, pâté 180
maksapasteija (Finnish pâté) 179
mayonnaise 196
meatballs, turkey, in tomato
  sauce 135
Mima's cabbage soup 66
motivation 8
Mrs H. S. Ball's chutney 112, 209
muffins, carrot and beetroot 170
mushroom
  soup, Thai 78
  sauce 128
mustard 196
  and anchovy dressing 192

noodles, Konnyaku 209
Nordic walking 20
'now to wow' lasagne 157

ohraryynipuuro (barley porridge)
  37
oils 209
onions, stuffed 112
pak choi stir-fry 187

pancakes
  banana 40
  courgette and bacon 41
pasta
  Bolognese, chilli 158
  ham and garlic, creamy 162
pâté
  Finnish (maksapasteija) 179
  salmon, creamy 180
  smoked mackerel 180
pea and mint soup 75
peanut dipping sauce 60
'pick me up' juice, purple 52
pizza, Turkish 114
planning 22
pomegranate
  and beef casserole 108
  molasses 209
pork sausage soup
  (siskonmakkarakeitto) 87
porridge
  barley (ohraryynipuuro) 37
  whipped, Finnish (vispipuuro)
    51
Portuguese squid 123
prawn(s)
  on bread (skagen) 38
  risotto, creamy 125
  stir-fry 126
prediabetes 7
protein bars, granola 173
purple 'pick me up' juice 52

quesadillas
  spinach and feta 63

raspberry smoothie 46
rice, chicken fried 134
rice paper rolls, seafood 60
Riche restaurant, Stockholm 38
risotto, creamy prawn 125
rogan josh, lamb 111
rooibos and apple iced tea 200
Russian soup (solyanka) 84

salad dressings

blueberry 96
mustard and anchovy 192
seafood 103
sushi 100
Waldorf 95
salads 95–103, 189
  halloumi, warm 96
  high fibre 189
  sushi 100
  Tex-Mex 98
  Waldorf 95
salmon
  pâté, creamy 180
  dill-cured salmon tartare 58
salsa, Tex-Mex 98
sangria, white wine 203
sauces see also dipping sauces
  mushroom 128
  sweet and sour 147
  tomato 135
sausage
  soup, pork
    (siskonmakkarakeitto) 87
  stew, vegetarian 146
scrambled eggs with caviar 48
seafood
  rice paper rolls 60
  salad 103
siskonmakkarakeitto (pork
  sausage soup) 87
skagen (prawns on bread) 38
sleep disorders 7
slow plan 10, 14–15, 27–9
smoked mackerel pâté 180
smoking 6
smoothie, raspberry 46
snacks, generally 165
solyanka (Russian soup) 84
soups 64–91 see also Filler Soups
  borscht 81
  cabbage, Mima's 66
  celeriac mushroom 71
  celery Roquefort 76
  chicken, Chinese 90
  chorizo, creamy 83
  fish 88

generally 57
leek and potato 91
mushroom, Thai 78
pea and mint 75
pork sausage
   (siskonmakkarakeitto) 87
Russian (solyanka) 84
side dishes for 63
summer 64
tom yum 67
tomato 72
tricolour 79
soya, light
cappuccino 207
latte 207
spicy chicken tacos 133
spinach and feta quesadilla 63
squid, Portuguese 123
stevia 209
stew
bacon and halloumi 117
cowboy 106
vegetarian sausage 146
stir-fry
pak choi 187
prawn 126
sweet and sour 147
stuffed onions 112
sumac 209
summer soup 64
sushi salad 100
sweet and sour stir-fry 147

Tabasco dip 176
tacos, spicy chicken 133
tahini paste 209
tea, iced
Earl Grey, with mint 199
rooibos and apple 200
Tex-Mex
salad 98
Thai mushroom soup 78
tobacco 6
tom yum soup 67
tomato
sauce 135

soup 72
tricolour soup 79
trout, baked 129
turkey
burgers with celeriac chips 130
meatballs in tomato sauce 135
Turkish pizza 114
turnip and celeriac bake 155

ultimate health loaf 174

vegetable
fajitas 150
green curry 152
vegetarian sausage stew 146
vispipuuro (Finnish whipped
   porridge) 51

Waldorf salad 95
warm halloumi salad 96
wasabi 209
whipped porridge, Finnish
   (vispipuuro) 51
white wine sangria 203
Wretman, Tore 38

yellow dal 149

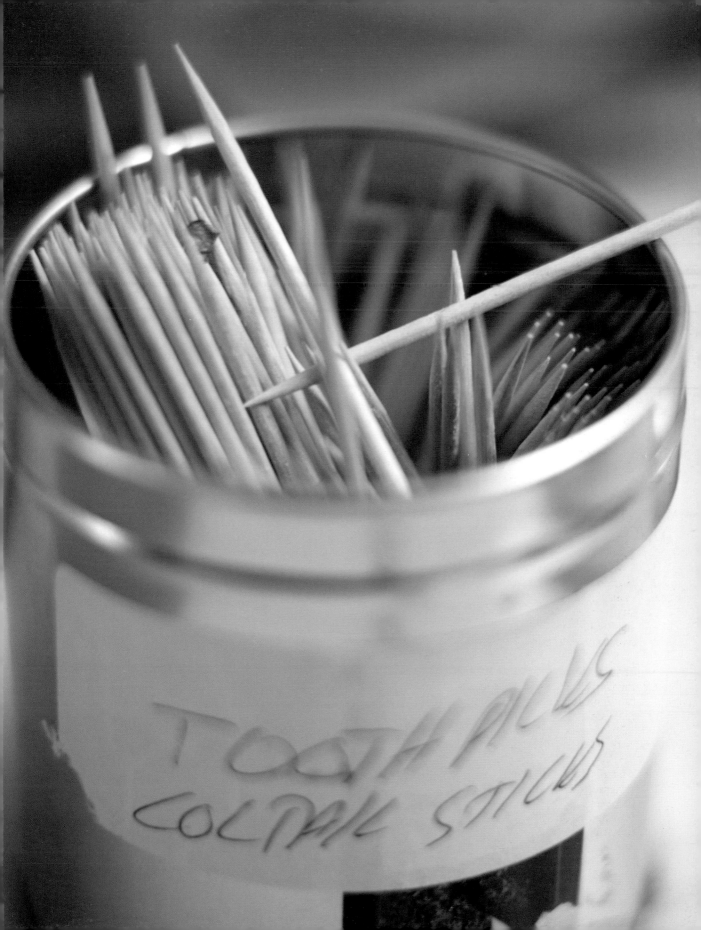